Seeing Christ in Sickness and Health

Peter Selg

Seeing Christ
in Sickness and Health

*Anthroposophical medicine as
a medicine founded in Christianity*

Floris Books

Translated by Christian von Arnim

First published in German under the title
Krankheit und Christus-Erkenntnis
by Verlag am Goetheanum, 2001
First published in English in 2005 by Floris Books

British Library CIP Data available

ISBN 0-86315-477-8

Produced by Polskabooks, Poland

For Dr Helene von Grunelius

August 14, 1897 – December 17, 1936

Unless otherwise noted, all translations from the New Testament are from Jon Madsen, *The New Testament*, Floris Books 1994. Those biblical passages marked RSV are from the Revised Standard Version.

Where the endnotes are more than textual references the endnote number is followed by an asterisk (*).

Contents

During a serious illness, one patient was fortunate enough to have Dr Helene von Grunelius as his physician. She frequently entered the sickroom in which he lay in a semi-conscious state. Quietly, without asking questions or speaking, she sat at his bedside, observing the patient. For the latter her presence was profoundly refreshing. The semi-conscious state of the patient was illuminated by a new will to live. It grew bright within him and a deep feeling of peace quelled the fever.

Whenever Helene von Grunelius was present, the patient felt himself strengthened in soul and body. It was as if she had given him food and drink of the finest sort which he was able to experience as physical nourishment.

Her nature allowed for no paralysing fear, no matter how serious the state of the patient. She was filled with the will to help. Patients were able to experience the devoted sacrificial willingness to take on the illness of her fellow human being in order to overcome it.

In a simple, wholly objective attitude of fellowship, she loved the human being in the person on which she exercised her medical skills on the basis of Christian illumination.

In Helene von Grunelius the beginnings of a new science of medicine were revealed which drew its capacity to help not just from sound medical knowledge, but which was accompanied by spiritual powers which she consciously mastered in Christian devotion.

This was particularly evident from the patient's perspective. The loss we experience at her death is great, but the knowledge to have encountered a human being of the future sublimates such loss into a life-affirming force.[1]

Preface

Peter Selg has dedicated this book on anthroposophical medicine to the physician Helene von Grunelius, who placed her life in the service of a medical practice which draws its inspiration from the personal search for and encounter with Christ. She died unexpectedly at the age of 39.

Although the phrase 'medicine founded in Christianity' may sound challenging, it nevertheless represents the most basic attribute of human fellowship which medicine and patient care can possess. The associated quality of warmth and confidence can be directly experienced by the reader of these studies. After all, it resides in and between the words written by Selg about medical practice founded in Christianity, and setting out its attitude and nature, its search for the correct path, and its willingness to act. A child psychiatrist by profession, it has become a particular concern of Peter Selg's to illustrate with spiritual empathy the path pursued by great medical personalities. In this book, he describes the 'inner physician' to whom Paracelsus refers, to the divine power of the higher self in the human being, to the meaning of St Paul's saying: 'Not I, but Christ in me.'

This book is aimed primarily at all those people who provide assistance to their sick fellow human beings as part of their daily work — nurses and carers, social workers and special needs teachers, therapists, ministers and physicians. They will find things presented here which belong to the intimate substance of the search on the inner path which can only be experienced meditatively. But this book can also provide valuable insights to the reader with a general interest in anthroposophy, insights about the objectives of a medicine which takes the inner spiritual core of the human being into account and thus has a primarily salutogenetic (health promoting) effect. Many of the sayings and meditations quoted here, as well as the illustrations included, produce something of their healing effect simply by being read.

Readers not familiar with anthroposophy will nevertheless understand the key elements from the context, particularly as the text is provided with full commentaries and support in the form of references.

Having published his comprehensive basic work, *Vom Logos menschlicher Physis* (On the Logos of human physis), followed by historical and biographical studies relating to anthroposophical medicine, it is now his endeavour to set out the characteristics of a medicine founded in Christianity which the science-based medicine of our time requires as a necessary complement.

Michaela Glöckler
Medical Section at the Goetheanum
Easter 2001

Introduction

*If you have really understood the spirit of
anthroposophy, you will find that anthroposophy in
turn opens the human ear and heart and the human
soul as a whole to the mystery of Christ. It is the
aim of the destiny of anthroposophy to coincide with
the destiny of Christianity.'*

Rudolf Steiner[1]

Anthroposophical medicine, established by Rudolf Steiner
(1861–1925) at the start of the twentieth century, saw and
sees itself explicitly as medicine founded in Christianity. It
began in 1921 with its first two clinics and from that time
onwards pursued its therapeutic course. Many of the
patients treated during the past eight decades in the spirit
of anthroposophical medicine felt that they were taken
seriously as individuals, that the specific biographical circumstances of their destiny were recognized and supported in a humane way — something which was
frequently put down to the apparently selfless ethics of
'anthroposophists' and was not further questioned. In
contrast, the intrinsic relationship between these positive
experiences and the spiritual sphere of the gospels was
seldom recognized, and sometimes studiously ignored
because of religious ties. Anthroposophical medicine, in
turn, neglected clearly to reveal its genuine Christian
basis, particularly in the context of its secondary literature,
and Rudolf Steiner himself did not hold a medical course
which overtly dealt with the subject.

But much in our present time depends on anthroposophical-based medicine going back to its roots and learning to make them accessible to people whose search — often born out of spiritual need and sometimes poorly articulated — will otherwise end in failure. Because the field of medicine has never been as confusing as now: physical medicine — single-mindedly dedicated to the paradigms of natural science and technology and engaged in an unstoppable dynamic which sweeps everything else before it — is contrasted by the hosts of alternative therapies whose confusing variety appears to promise an answer to everything. How are we to find a path through all these things which is human? Human in the sense of the person who rightly perceives his illness as individual destiny, whose requirement for treatment does not exhaust itself in physiological normalization or psychotherapeutic life analysis, and who frequently is searching for concepts which have a greater basis in spirituality than is normally available. For the encounter with illness has always been connected with the mystery of a person's own incarnation and throws up profound questions, even if they do not always reach the full light of consciousness.

What distinguishes anthroposophical medicine is that it poses these questions in a radical way, opening up a fundamental perspective on the nature of the human being, as even its critics will sometimes admit. But contrary to what is widely imputed, the knowledge of the human being set out by anthroposophy is not based on the teachings of eastern wisdom, but is a genuinely western science of the spirit with a Christian focus. Understanding this connection more profoundly does not lead to some — historically long obsolete — rhapsody about European preeminence, but to a recognition of the basis in the history of ideas of Steiner's works and their spiritual distinction. *Et incarnatus est:* the incarnation of Christ in a human body at that turning-point in history was the beginning of a healing current in the evolution of the earth and human beings; with a view to the continuing influence of this turning-point in world history, Rudolf Steiner at the start of the twentieth century formulated what he called anthroposophical medicine.

The essays in this book set out different but related aspects of anthroposophical medicine as a medicine founded in Christianity. They were written in response to individual questions and issues which led me to an intensive study of Rudolf Steiner's statements as well as his fundamental medical and therapeutic objectives. That is how these studies came to be written. They illustrate the immense focus on Christ of Rudolf Steiner's work as much as the importance of individual medical personalities among his followers. Their remembrance supported me in writing this book — above all Ita Wegman (1876–1943), Helene von Grunelius (1897–1936) and Gerhard Kienle (1923–83).

The first chapter, 'Et Incarnatus Est' considers the accounts of healing in the New Testament on the basis of anthroposophy and sets out the therapeutic processes which come to bear in them. Rudolf Steiner's medical initiative as a whole must be seen against this archetypal background. This can be clearly seen in the structure and the historical circumstances of his medical works as much as in Steiner's consultative therapeutic activity in the surgeries of the anthroposophical doctors learning from him.

The next chapter, 'From Empathy with Suffering to Karmic Resolve,' illustrates how Rudolf Steiner intended to re-establish the Christian therapeutic resolve in the spirit of the Gospel of Luke among physicians, nurses and other therapists. Such a therapeutic attitude, described by Steiner as a series of stages, applies to *everyone* working in the medical field; in terms of its content it is not restricted to a feeling of empathy with the patient, although such a feeling provides the irreplaceable and continuing basis for all therapeutic endeavours of assistance. In the final analysis, the cognition and resolve of the attending physician is affected at an existential level — a soul and spiritual process which must currently be undertaken amidst an intense spiritual conflict increasingly threatening the medical field and, indeed, trying to extinguish its healing endeavours. Few people in the twentieth century saw this as clearly as the physician Gerhard Kienle who in the spirit of Rudolf Steiner made every attempt to preserve the social effectiveness of medicine founded in Christianity.

The third chapter, 'The Healing Medicine,' investigates the relationship between the sacrament of communion — the real accomplishment of transubstantiation — and medicine. That there do exist inner spiritual links between both spheres which have their foundation in the comprehensive work of Christ and which extend into the processes of physical substance has undoubtedly been experienced repeatedly in the western history of ideas. But it has been clearly formulated only in a rudimentary way — most impressively by Paracelsus in the sixteenth century. Four hundred years later, Rudolf Steiner's medical and theological works developed new and future-oriented perspectives on the basis of epistemological methodology which should not be ignored by a future medicine serving the needs of people.

The concluding fourth chapter about the human heart as an organ of destiny ('The soul quickens in the shrine of the heart'), illustrates by means of examples the spiritual and Christological background of anthroposophical human physiology. In terms of its innermost composition, but also in terms of its functionality, the human body — 'the conclusion of the paths of God' as Oetinger described it — is one of the open secrets which continues to be misjudged, leading to sustained consequences for civilization. It is no accident that a meditation by Rudolf Steiner for his closest collaborator in the medical field, the physician Ita Wegman, forms the heart of this small study. The collaboration between Steiner and Wegman produced a direction in medicine whose aim is to be to incorporate a future-oriented medicine founded in Christianity into the 'mystery of the earth.'[2]

This book is dedicated to the memory of the anthroposophical physician Helene von Grunelius, who died at a young age. She formed the 'soul' of a group of medical students, linked by destiny, who approached Rudolf Steiner in their search of a truly human-oriented medical practice and who received concentrated instruction from him. The intensive way in which Helene von Grunelius was able to make use of this for herself is shown by the experience of the patient whose report is set at the start of this book. May these 'beginnings of a new science of medicine' continue under the conditions of the twenty-first century — through all those people who make it their endeavour.

My thanks are due to the publisher at the Goetheanum, Joseph Morel, whose warm and great enthusiasm made this book possible. They are also due to the many listeners who supported and responded so positively to the original lectures. Their sustained interest gave me the courage to publish these studies, which in the strictest sense remain provisional in nature.

Peter Selg
Kirchhofen, Freiburg
Easter 2001

1. Et Incarnatus Est

Healing in the Gospels and the Medicine of Rudolf Steiner

I have not come not to judge human beings, but to heal them.

John 12:47

And he wandered through all Galilee and taught in the synagogues there and proclaimed the message of salvation from the heavenly world and healed all the illnesses and infirmities from which the people suffered. Soon he was spoken about in the whole of Syria and they brought to him all who were ill with many kinds of disease, those who were suffering, those possessed, somnabulists and those who were paralysed, and he healed them all.

Matt.4:23f

At the start of the third Christian millennium and at the end of the first century of anthroposophical medicine, it appears appropriate to examine once more the accounts of healing in the gospels. If we take into consideration that according to Rudolf Steiner the future task of Central Europe is connected essentially with the development of therapeutic, healing faculties, an understanding of the

Im gefühle der Bedürftigkeit DEINER gnade,
Christus-Licht der Welt, harre ich
    nach Kräften
    öffnend der Seele Pforten

  DEINER Erleuchtung
Still in mir will ich sein
und DIR danken DEINER gabe
und sie geben
als DEIN Geschenk an Menschen
Werkzeug DEINES Wortes
will ich sein
mit meiner Seele
    besten Kräften
    echten Tiefen
    stillsten Erfurchten.

Page from Rudolf Steiner's notebook (undated)

concrete healing activity of Jesus Christ takes on a key significance, an almost founding significance for the position
of the Christian West, at least from the perspective of
anthroposophy. We will therefore attempt to develop
some key aspects related to healing in the gospels and to
show in what respect the new medicine inaugurated by
Rudolf Steiner in the twentieth century has an inner connection to them.

The Christ of the gospels came to earth as the 'Saviour.'
Even the name of Jesus denotes the 'spiritual physician' in
a Middle Eastern language, according to Steiner.[1] *Sozein,*
the process of healing, expressly penetrates all four
gospels in a broad sweep and in individual, concrete
descriptions of events. But in German Martin Luther and
later in English the King James translation rendered the
Greek verb as 'saved,' thus introducing the fatal process of
a mere psychological interpretation of the accounts of
Christ healing the sick. When we read: 'and the Son of
Man has come to seek and to save what was lost' (Luke
19:10), it means that the close physical attention paid by
Jesus Christ to those people he found sick and in need is
relegated into the dim background, thus also relegating to
forgetfulness a central profound dimension of his being —
a being which truly incarnated and connected with its
physical environment.

But Christ *healed* the earth and the many individual people who encountered him with their physical sufferings —
the New Testament reports about it in vividly recorded
documents. To those individuals and their cure there
accrues wide-reaching, almost archetypal and symbolic
significance. Wee see this, for instance, when Christ, whose
'I' is the 'light of the world,' was able to heal the blind —
those who were born blind and those who became blind —

and make them see again; or when he, the cosmic Word, gave back language to the deaf and dumb man.[2]

The key significance of the therapeutic medical mission of Christ can also be seen in the sending out into the world of the close circle of his pupils, the disciples. They were to carry his Logos — the Word — into the world *and* heal the sick. They were often present when Christ healed the sick and on occasion were very specifically included in the healing process, as for example the disciples Peter, James and John in the healing of Jairus' daughter. That his pupils were at least partially on the right track is made clear in the gospels through the reference that the disciples — to their considerable own surprise — really did manage to achieve independent healing processes.[3] Jesus Christ was able to transfer his powers of healing to them at least partially 'because of their particular karma.'[4]

If, on the other hand, the disciples did not succeed in their therapeutic activity in individual instances — for example in the case of the sick boy at the foot of Mount Tabor — Christ reacted almost with annoyance. In Rudolf Steiner's translation it says in Luke 9:41: 'How weak is the inner power of faith in you ... [I must] remain with you and bear with you *for some time yet until your powers can also stream into the other people.*'[5] Here Jesus Christ acted with his healing powers on behalf of the unsuccessful disciples and helped the boy. However, Christ's final healing of the sick in the New Testament is that of Malchus the soldier whose ear had been injured by one of the disciples, Peter. Thus even at the end Christ still *healed* the failure of one of his first disciples.

Malchus was healed through the *touch* of Christ: 'And he touched the ear and healed him' (Luke 22:51). If we look

as a whole at the acts of healing which Christ undertook
— even just in the outward description of the four evan-
gelists — there are various concrete methods of healing or
forms of therapeutic intervention which must be distin-
guished from one another, and which represent a
sequence of therapeutic incarnations of the Logos. Christ
frequently healed solely through the action of his *word*,
spoken with full authority and power, with Exousiai and
Dynameis, the 'I AM' *(ego eimi)* whose profound force right
down to a physical level was felt even by the soldiers pur-
suing him into the garden of Gethsemane: 'Now when he
said to them: I AM he, they reeled back and fell to the
ground.' (John 18:6) But sick people of good will were
healed by his word, it lifted them up in contrast to the soldiers who fell to the ground.

In various acts of healing Christ's word was then rein-
forced through a guiding or, indeed, a threatening *gesture*,
as when demons are driven out for example. Then there
are healing processes which are introduced by a linguistic
command from Christ to the sick person — a command to
act through the ego and with intent. The man with the
withered hand had to extend it, others had to get up from
their bed or start to move themselves — and were healed.

Then, as in the case of the soldier Malchus, numerous
instances of a concrete *touch* by Christ are described. Such
touching took the form of the laying on of a hand or of
hands, including the laying of Christ's hands on the eyes
of the blind man or the finger of Christ in the ears of the
deaf man. An intensification of such physical closeness
takes place in the moistening of the tongue (deaf man) or
the eyes (blind man) with Christ's own saliva.

Finally there is a last spiritual and physical culmination, what might be described as a preliminary form of

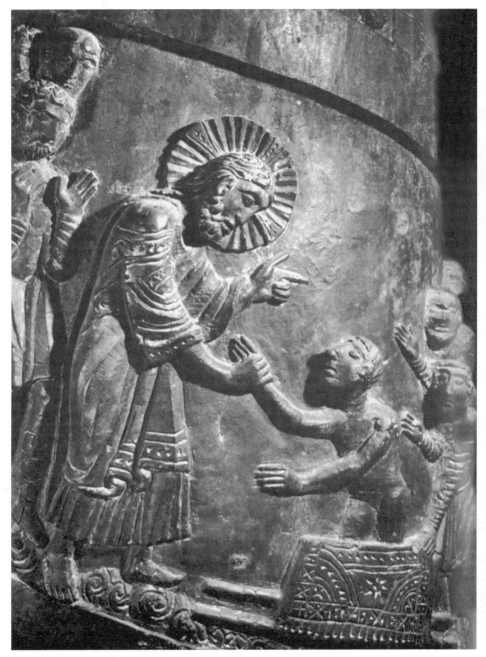

The raising of the young man at Nain (Hildesheim, c. 1000)

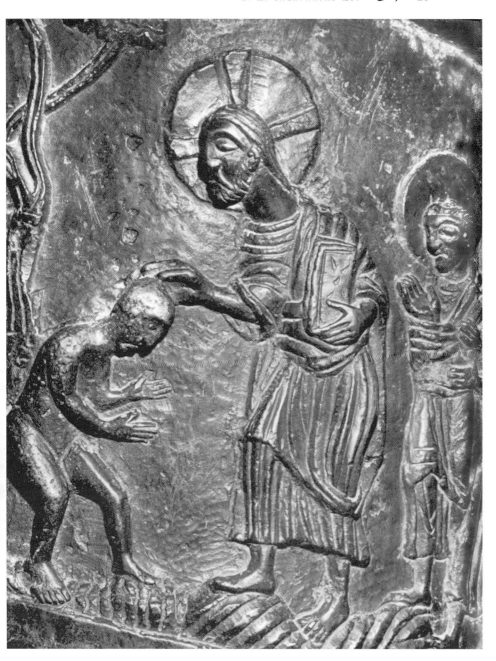

The healing of the leper (Hildesheim, c. 1000)

material transubstantiation, when Christ's saliva is mixed with the earth, creating a paste which was laid on the blind eyes of the sick man.

The healing processes briefly described here — from the healing word to the spiritualized substance of the earth, via heat, air and water — once again reflect the actual movement of incarnation of the being of Christ from heaven to earth: *Et incarnatus est,* 'And the Word became flesh, and lived among us.' (John 1:14) The being of Christ took hold of the earth with healing intent; it penetrated the body of Jesus, had a direct and substantive effect on its environment and, finally, completely united itself with the earth as a whole.

> When we ... look at the New Testament, it is striking how many acts of healing there are. ... If we consider this, we might conclude that the New Testament represents the inauguration of a medical or socio-medical movement: the poor are fed, the poor are looked after and the sick are healed.[6]

The medical 'inauguration' sketched out in the gospels was given only a very qualified reception and continuation in the West, essentially restricted to spiritually deepened nursing care.[7] There were only few exceptions such as Paracelsus (1493–1541) who, wholly grounded in the gospels and esoteric Christianity, was able to exercise powers of healing and proclaim the Word (see p. 86ff.). In fact, the archetypal medical and therapeutic concern of the New Testament lived and survived the post-medieval centuries in the spiritual sphere of the Rosicrucians before being thoroughly resurrected in Rudolf Steiner's anthroposophical medicine at the end of the second Christian millennium.

'Having stood in spirit before the mystery of Golgotha

in the most intimate and serious celebration of compre-
hension was a key element in my soul development,'
Steiner wrote at the end of his life in characterizing the
course of his destiny and the development of his cognition
shortly before the turn of the century.[8]*

In 1902, he turned for the first time to the subject of the
raising of Lazarus in his book about *Christianity as Mystical
Fact*. Soon after, he began a medical collaboration with the
theosophical physician Ludwig Noll in Kassel, and thus in
the city in which Steiner gave early lectures on the Rosicrucians and the Gospel of St John. The last lecture cycle
given by him in September 1924 was a pastoral-medical
course for anthroposophical physicians and the priests of
the newly-established Christian Community. It reached its
conclusion in the formulation of the healing mantra, 'I will
walk the path.'[9] One person who attended the course, Dr
Madeleine van Deventer, subsequently wrote: 'The mystery character shone through and culminated in the concluding lecture about the renewal of the mysteries in a
profoundly Christian sense.'[10]

In the very last period of his work, Steiner still established the esoteric core of the Medical Section and thus a
real 'Raphael School' whose members were ceremoni-
ously inducted before the statue of Christ in the Dornach
studio.[11] The beginning and end of Steiner's medical lec-
turing activity was wholly marked by a spiritually profound understanding of Christ, of which he experienced
the healing effectiveness.

> Up to the fourth cultural period, in which Christ
> appeared and in which there were still sufficient
> numbers of people in whom one could see how
> the spirit could affect the physical, humankind

gradually ... lost the ability of the soul and spirit
to control the physical. Christ had to appear that
time. Had he come later none of the things which
were shown at that time could have been shown.
Such a major phenomenon had to enter the world,
and it did so just in time.[12]

According to Rudolf Steiner, the human constitution was
considerably different at the time of the events in the
gospels from the present situation — the human incarnation process, the process of a profound connection
between the spirit and soul and the living physical element had not at that time reached its culmination. At the
time of Christ there was — as in previous periods but in a
weaker form — a certain independence of the life body
from the physical organization. The powerful etheric
body, Steiner says, extended beyond the physical organism controlled by it; the physical body itself was still soft,
malleable and sensitive.

Such an overall constitution of the human being
enabled not just elementary spiritual perception but also
facilitated soul and spiritual processes strongly affecting
the life processes: 'The human body at that time was still
subject to a much greater, we might say immediate influence through the power of the soul, the power of the
spirit, than later when the body had become denser and
the soul as a result lost its power over the body.'[13] With the
human constitution in this kind of a state, healing
processes in a body which had fallen ill had to be undertaken via the soul; the latter, properly controlled, had the
ability to penetrate the body 'with the healing forces
fetched from the spiritual world if the body had become
disordered, so that such forces could enable the body to
restore its harmony and order.'

That is why at the time of the gospels there were still many physicians who were able to heal spiritually. The members of the Essene order, to whom Jesus had for a time stood close before the baptism in Jordan, were directly called 'therapists' in Egypt. Like many other people with such abilities, they worked with spiritual forces. 'They cleansed the soul and filled it with healthy feelings, impulses, and forces of will through soul and spiritual influences,' which in turn had an ordering effect on the confused physical situation of the sick person.[14*]

If the therapeutic activities of Jesus Christ were thus in certain respects connected with the traditions of spiritually-shaped healing processes in the ancient cultures, Rudolf Steiner nevertheless describes them as a fundamentally new event, as the signature of this 'turning point in history.' For in contrast to the pre-Christian healers trained in the medical mystery schools, who had developed themselves into receptive instruments of cosmic spiritual forces in dulling and, indeed, sacrificing their own ego consciousness, and thus affecting the sick person in a directly magical and mediumistic fashion, Christ radically worked on the basis of the forces of his 'I.'

In 1912, Rudolf Steiner said in Basle:

> The significant fact [of Christ's healing] is not that healing took place, but that someone appeared who was able to heal in this way without having been in a mystery school; that someone appeared who possessed in his own heart, his own soul the forces which previously had flowed from the higher worlds, and that these forces had become personal, individual forces.[15]

In Christ the heavenly forces had become individualized; he worked on the basis of the heart-forces of his world-encompassing self in which heaven had come down to earth — *et incarnatus est.*

Rudolf Steiner described the healing activity of Christ as a 'force of overflowing love' in his lectures on the Gospel of St Luke, also referring to it as 'love overflowing the dimension of the self.'[16] *Ex abundantia enim cordis os loquitor* (Matt.12:34): out of the abundance of the heart Christ's mouth spoke, from his radiating 'I' in the heart forces emanated the healing and holy powers. In the gospels this is indicated not least by the reference to major passions in the being of Christ just before the healing action. The 'weeping,' 'anger' or 'sighing' of Christ refers to an emotion of the self in the heart. Friedrich Rittelmeyer therefore translates the raising of Lazarus as: 'So he (Christ) welled up in the spirit. Body and soul shook.'[17]

Jesus Christ acted out of his 'I' and he worked on the 'I' of his sick interlocutor. Healing no longer took place magically, circumventing the individual will of the sick person. On the contrary, in order to be effective Christ required the affirmative volition, and thus the willingness to receive, of the other self: 'Your faith helped you!' It is also explicitly noted in the gospels that Christ was *only* able to heal in this way. In Nazareth, where he encountered little faith, there was no healing activity. It is the affirmative power of faith, grounded in the 'I,' which is described by Rudolf Steiner as being able to receive the Christ impulse in a person's own being or which can work *as the power of Christ* in a person's soul: 'Everyone has faith who receives Christ within himself, so that Christ can live in him, and his "I" is not just an empty vessel but overflows with content. And this overflowing content is none other than the content of love.'[18]

Through his 'I,' Christ works on the different levels of

being of the sick person which are affected. Using the individual examples of healing of the possessed man, the paralysed man as well as the woman with the flow of blood and the daughter of Jairus, Steiner shows how each of the illnesses occur at the level of the soul body (possessed man), life organism (paralysed man) and physical organization (woman and Jairus' daughter), something which we will not discuss here in detail.[19]* In various encounters with the sick, Christ also pointed to the karmic background of the illnesses he encountered, according to Steiner's explanations — as for example in healing the man born blind as well as raising the daughter of Jairus.[20]*

Christ's response to the question of his disciples as to the background of the suffering of the man born blind — generally translated as: 'It was not that this man sinned, or his parents, but that the works of God might be made manifest in him' (John 9:3 RSV) — is rendered by Steiner as: 'He was born blind so that the works of "God in him" could be made visible.' Explaining and expanding his rendering, he adds: 'Neither he nor his parents have sinned, he fulfils his karma so that the spark of God may become visible in him, so that the works of the "God in him" (that is, his eternal 'I') become visible.'[21] With regard to the twelve-year-old daughter of Jairus, Rudolf Steiner indicated a karmic relationship with the woman with the flow of blood — sick for twelve years — who is healed by Christ on his way to Jairus' house, and remarked: 'That is how deep we must enter into things to grasp the karma between people.'[22]

That Steiner here saw not just the *origin* of the course of various illnesses in the gospels in a karmic context, but also the nature and the *timing* of the healing intervention of Christ, is illustrated by a remark in his lectures on the

Gospel of St Mark in which he says: 'Jesus Christ thus stands at our side as a figure with enlightened insight into karma when he reveals: I can heal him because I can see from his personality that his karma is such that he may now rise and walk.'[23]*

'When in millennia human beings will have acquired what emanates as power from the Christ ego, then the human egos will be able to achieve effects which are the same as the ones projected by Christ into humanity at that time.'[24] The healing processes at the time of Christ also possess a future-oriented, anticipatory significance, according to Rudolf Steiner. Current humanity and the medical practice it requires are moving towards the increasing strengthening of the self, leading to the renewed dominance of the human spirit soul over the life organism; are moving towards a spirit soul, an existential force penetrated by the 'I,' which will in future be able to exercise an ordering influence wholly in the spirit of the gospels, for: 'The "I" will be such at the end of its development that it contains Christ in totality.'[25]

The maturing of the ego in the sick person as the result of the healing process triggered by Christ is expressed most forcefully in the healing of the man born blind in the Gospel of St John. Such ego development flows into a gradually enhanced understanding of Christ, as Rudolf Frieling was able to show in detail in a subtle reflection on the textual form of the gospel.[26] The blind man who has regained his sight embarks on the progressive development of his individuality in actively overcoming his illness which results in the loss of all traditional ties and the internalization of the power of the Christ within his self.

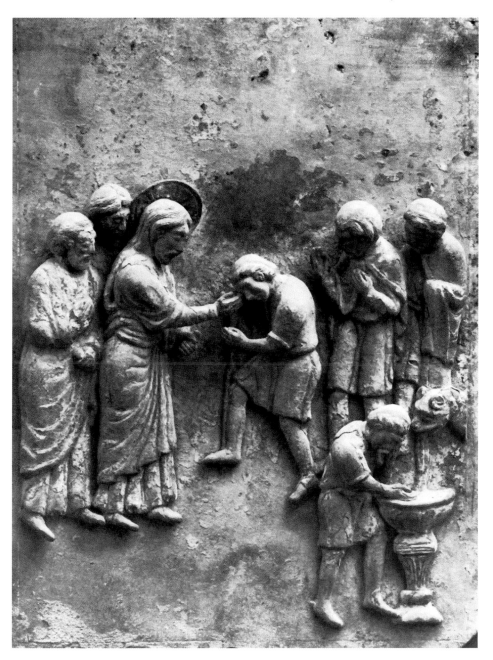

The healing of the man born blind (Benevent, c. 1150)

Finally he becomes capable of saying the words of Christ, 'I am,' himself.[27]* In this way the report in John ends in the blind man's cognition of Christ: 'Jesus heard that they had thrown him out [of the synagogue], and he found him and said to him, "Do you trust in the Son of Man?" He answered, "Tell me who he is, Lord, so that I may place my trust in him." Then Jesus said, "You have seen him. He it is who is speaking to you." And he said, "I believe, Lord." And he fell down before him.' (John 9:35–38). A short while later Christ uttered the great words: 'I AM the good shepherd, and I know who belongs to me; and those who are mine know me' (John 10:14).

'Then Jesus said,"You have seen him".' According to Rudolf Steiner, Christ became increasingly open to being perceived in the etheric sphere from 1909 onwards. At Whitsun 1912, Steiner for the first time spoke of the necessity — and, indeed, of the now soluble problem — of representing the figure of Christ in a truthful sculpture, ('as he really ... is'[28]) in lectures in Cologne (May 8) and Berlin (May 14). He described the face of Christ with the forehead in wondrous amazement, the eyes filled with empathy and a mouth from which the divine word flows faithfully. He said in Berlin among other things:

> Any depiction of Christ should actually represent something like the ideal figure of Christ. And this is the feeling we should develop as we endeavour to achieve such an ideal, that in increasing measure the following feeling must arise in human development when humankind undertakes artistic activity to represent the highest ideal through spiritual science: 'You must not look at what already exists when you wish to depict Christ, but

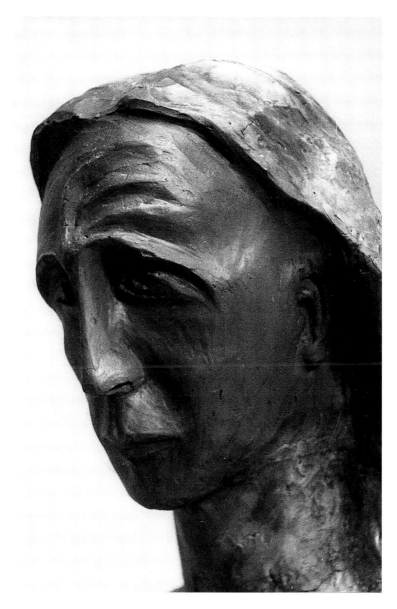

Side view of the sculpture of Christ by Rudolf Steiner (Dornach 1915)

you must allow to be active and work in you and
permit yourself to be penetrated by everything
you can acquire through spiritual contemplation
of the development of the world through the three
important impulses of wonder, empathy and con-
science.'[29]

In the autumn of 1914, the destined collaboration between
Rudolf Steiner and the English sculptress Edith Maryon
on the sculpture of Christ began in the Dornach studio.
This was to be the Goetheanum's crowning element of the
whole building — and the central image for a new medicine based in Christianity (compare p. 80).

Six months later, in the spring of 1915, the Protestant
theologian Friedrich Rittelmeyer sought out Rudolf
Steiner in Nuremberg for a meeting in which he wished to
discuss in greater depth his experience of strong physical
effects following meditation of Christ's sayings. In 1928,
looking back on that meeting, Rittelmeyer wrote:

It was as if these word (of Christ) said: if we are to
live in you, we must first refashion you. The intimate spiritual corporeality which stands behind
physical corporeality came to consciousness. It
created awareness of changes. The meditation of
the sayings of Christ could be intensified to produce strong physical feelings, indeed active physical pain. The subsequent experience was then one
of an overwhelming therapeutic awareness which
gave an inkling of what real health of the whole
human being means. This experience made me
wonder whether it was not possible to say something about Christ's real appearance on the basis
such meditation of Christ's words. One would
then have to observe with regard to certain limits

of one's own physicality in what respect Christ
must have been different from oneself. Christ's
words express more or less clearly what the body
must look like in which they could truly live. ...
Without going into these observations in detail, I
asked Rudolf Steiner: 'Is it actually possible to
reach a stage of being able to say something about
the appearance of Christ simply by meditating on
Christ's sayings?'[30]

In conversation, Steiner guided Rittelmeyer to the figure
of Christ as it had become visible and enabled him — in
the middle of the War — to follow the creation of the
wooden sculpture in Dornach: 'Thus at the time I experienced the gospels before this image of Christ.'[31] Friedrich
Rittelmeyer subsequently became the first head of the
Christian Community, a movement which received sustained support from Rudolf Steiner.

The first medical course, the beginning in the twentieth
century of a new medicine based on the individual, began
in the spring of 1920 in Steiner's Dornach studio — in
proximity to the figure of Christ.[32*] The conversation
between Rudolf Steiner and the young Dutch physician
Willem Zeylmans van Emmichoven on colours and the
etheric also took place in the same place at Christmas
1920: 'Yes, that is Christ as my spiritual eye perceived him
in Palestine,' Steiner told the surprised Zeylmans, introducing him to the etheric language of forms and thus into
the sphere of medicine and the new revelation of Christ in
the twentieth century.[33]

A further six months later, in the early summer of 1921,
Rudolf Steiner began his consultations in Ita Wegman's
clinic in Arlesheim. Steiner saw patients, described the
layer of their being and the karmic background of their

illness, then prescribed specific medicines, applications, artistic exercises and meditations which were intended to stimulate ego activity: Steiner practiced a new medicine whose archetype and active model was the future-oriented medicine of the gospels. In the autumn of 1923, he gave the young physician Helene von Grunelius the meditation 'How can I find what is good' — an exercise for the perception of Christ in the etheric which was intended to prepare esoterically the group of medical friends connected in destiny with Helene von Grunelius for the task of penetrating medicine with Christ.[34]

A short time later (in October 1923), Steiner's joint work with Ita Wegman began in the studio near the sculpture of Christ on the manuscript which finally was to result in the book *Fundamentals of Therapy*. The project was marked by the Lord's Prayer which Rudolf Steiner spoke as an introduction to the work which began every evening at about six o'clock.[35] According to Emil Bock, this hour when the *spiritual* day began — the time when worship takes place in the Old Testament and in Islam — was also the hour in which Christ in the Gospel of St Mark began his great healing activity on the Sea of Galilee: 'It was already getting late, the sun was setting, and they brought to him all who were sick and possessed' (Mark 1:32).

Finally, Rudolf Steiner also received three young people in the Christ studio during Christmas 1923 who asked him about the destiny of disabled children and how to help them. Albrecht Strohschein, Siegfried Pickert and Franz Löffler took what Steiner told them deep into their heart and established anthroposophical special needs education with the support of Steiner and Wegman, in which a hidden 'stream of anthroposophical life' which was a direct part of esoteric Christianity became directly visible.[36]

If the key stages in the genesis of the new anthroposophical medicine took place under such express Christological prerequisites, if the whole of its diction — developed in an exemplary way in the visits to Arlesheim and practiced in the various therapeutic institutions — was aimed at supporting the individual and his destiny, then the concrete spiritual relationship of the medicine inaugurated by Rudolf Steiner with the therapeutic processes described in the New Testament was revealed not least in the individual meditative exercises which Steiner gave to sick people. In these exercises, the power of Christ's Logos took effect in a way cautiously entrusted to the ill person, given to him in freedom; in other words, made subject to his active will. We will conclude this outline by referring in particular to two therapeutic meditations which Rudolf Steiner gave to a child and a dying person.

The first exercise was given to a ten-year-old Stuttgart schoolboy who had injured his eye. Rudolf Steiner prescribed internal medicines, specific compresses for the eye and then he wrote the following meditative words on the prescription pad, reading them out aloud as he wrote them:

> The stars shine
> It is night
> Peace fills this room
> There is silence
> I feel the peace
> I feel the silence
> In my heart
> In my head
> God speaks Christ speaks.

KLINISCH-THERAPEUTISCHES INSTITUT
STUTTGART
GANSHEIDESTRASSE 88 / TELEPHON 1189

Rezept für ....

....

Es scheinen die Sterne

Es ist Nacht

Es füllt Ruhe den Raum

alles schweigt

Ich fühle die Ruhe

Ich fühle das Schweigen

In meinem Herzen

In meinem Kopf

Stuttgart, den..

Gott spricht Christus spricht.

Verse written by Rudolf Steiner (1924)

Half a year later at Epiphany of 1925, the year in which Rudolf Steiner died, this child, who later became an anthroposophical physician, was led by Ita Wegman to his sick bed in the Dornach studio:

I had to walk a few feet alone through the room. The walk seemed to take infinitely long. The mighty wooden sculpture stood there, attracting the eye. Rudolf Steiner's bed was positioned in front of this statue of Christ. The closer I approached, the more ceremonious and great this last encounter became. Rudolf Steiner sat up in bed and looked at me with eyes which radiated an indescribable love. The physical room disappeared and a wide space was created, accompanied by radiating warmth. I can no longer remember what was said. Then he laid his hand on my head and spoke the words which have stayed with me since: 'It is good.'[37]

It was an act of blessing which confirmed and concluded the healing process.[38]*

The second exercise was entrusted by Rudolf Steiner to a person who was dying. Six months before she died, Rudolf Steiner said with reference to the woman suffering from cancer:

She should imagine every evening that she is walking up a high mountain and when she has reached the top she should imagine seeing Christ coming towards her from the other side saying to her: 'Receive my strength.' She should thoroughly experience these words in her heart and in the morning she should recall this meditation like a prayer.[39]

The nocturnal stars of the cosmos shone for the growing child, while the sun power of Christ came towards the dying woman. Thus the new age of a human, Christian medicine began.

2. From Empathy with Suffering to Karmic Resolve

Stages of a Therapeutic Intention

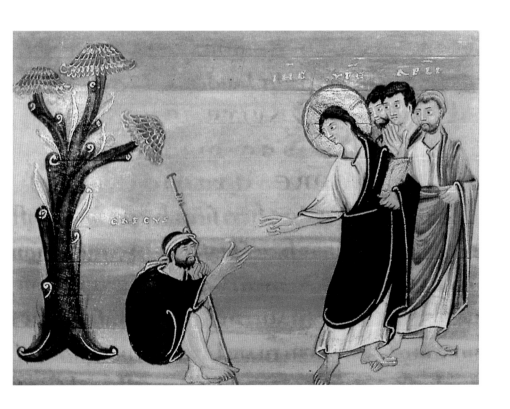

The healing of the blind man (Codex Egberti, c. 980)

I will mention one case here which deeply impressed me. A patient fell ill with peritonitis accompanied by a high temperature. The clinical picture became so ominous that experienced colleagues abandoned any hope. Dr Wegman spent three days and nights almost exclusively at the bedside of the patient; two junior doctors and two nurses assisted her. Therapeutic measures were continuously carried out, mostly by her: the racked body was lightly massaged with etheric oils, enemas administered and injections given, sips of champagne fed. The atmosphere in the room was almost unbearable and felt 'laden with demons' The younger helpers among us found it difficult to keep going and were frequently sent out by her to refresh ourselves in the garden. We felt somewhat ashamed to see that Dr Wegman did not need to be relieved. After three days the worst was over, the temperature returned to normal and nutrition became possible again. The patient returned to full health — albeit after a lengthy convalescence.

Madeleine van Deventer[1]

From the beginning, Rudolf Steiner wished to have the Goetheanum as a *site of knowledge* accompanied by a *site of healing.* Spiritual scientific research was to lead to social action for the benefit of the sick and people in need — as had been the case in the ancient spiritual cultures. The central focus, indeed, the crowning element of the Goetheanum was to be a sculpture of Christ: Christ between the adversary powers of Lucifer and Ahriman, illustration of a new science based in Christianity, a Michaelic and Christian Aristotelianism.[2*] It is no great leap to assume that this sculpture, which was to form the central focus of the School of Spiritual Science, was also intended to become the core image of the new anthroposophical medicine.

But if we study the transcripts which have been preserved of Steiner's 'intellectual' medical courses (Ita Wegman[3*]) there is, on a superficial level, hardly any mention of a 'medicine based in Christianity,' of Christ or, indeed, of the forces that oppose the divine. On the contrary, they are dominated by descriptions introducing a new physiological, pathophysiological and therapeutic *thinking* and showing how such therapy can be methodologically developed from an understanding of the illness. Was this the foundation of a new medicine based in Christianity?

There is only *one* place in his medical lectures where Rudolf Steiner — in response to a question — refers directly to the necessity to imbue medicine with Christianity, and that is at Easter 1924 speaking to numerous medical students and selected physicians. He categorically pointed out to these young people, who had asked for particular guidance in their medical and therapeutic training, that in terms of the history of ideas current scientific orthodox medicine taught at university should be seen as an 'alien body' within European and western civilization. It contained no original 'Christian will to heal' since it originated in the Arab world and had received its particular and still effective character there. In this context Rudolf Steiner described the future reception of the Gospel of St Luke as essential for the training of corresponding therapeutic abilities.[4]

In his own lectures on Luke's 'gospel of healing' Steiner had said as early as fifteen years previously (1909) that the therapeutic capacity of Christ was a 'power of overflowing love.' Christ, the incarnated cosmic Logos, had such great love in him, Steiner said, overflowing and abundant to such an extent that it 'overflowed to all those around him who wanted to regain their health.'[5] At Whitsun of the following year (1910), Rudolf Steiner in the specifically medical Hamburg lectures on the formation and transformation of destiny, *The Manifestation of Karma,* then developed in greater detail precisely this dimension of love in the therapeutic encounter and action ('We take the medicine either from the environment, from the densified light, or from our own soul, from the healing act of love, act of sacrifice, and then heal with the soul power acquired from love'[6]). But these connections, set out in a memorable way in Hamburg in 1910 and repeated again in the gospel cycles, were evidently only understood to a limited degree by Steiner's listeners and not recognized in their fundamental medical and therapeutic significance. The medical movement which Steiner hoped would arise in the small theosophical group of physicians did not come about at the time — and thus the subject of the 'Christian will to heal' also continued largely to rest.[7*]

Nevertheless, Steiner's later accounts, occurring in parallel with the development of the concepts of *experience of suffering, sense of helping, will to heal, courage to heal* and *karmic resolve,* appear as the finely differentiated echo of this motif of therapeutic Christian love. With extreme caution it appears occasionally in the medical courses and yet is at work in the background of Steiner's accounts, setting their hidden tone.

Experience of suffering, sense of helping, will to heal, courage to heal and *karmic resolve* describe the soul and spiritual path of a medicine based in Christianity and the path of the Christian therapist. They form the basic concepts of a new medicine and lead to that figure which Rudolf Steiner created from autumn 1914 onwards in many years of collaboration with Edith Maryon and before whose visage he accepted the first members into the new medical mystery school in September 1924.

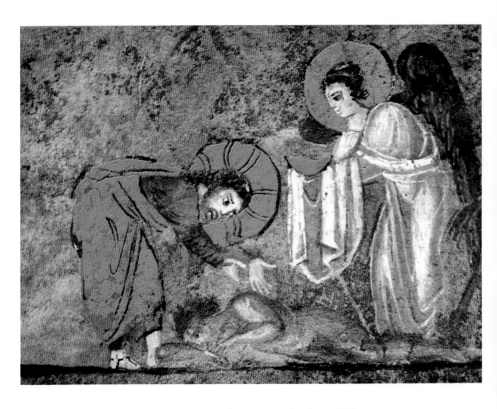

Christ as the Good Samaritan (Syria, c. 550)

From empathy with suffering
to the courage to heal

As long as you *feel the pain*
Which does not affect me
Christ remains unrecognized
At work in cosmic existence;
For the spirit remains weak
If it can feel suffering
In its own body alone.
                    Rudolf Steiner[8]

This meditative verse was given by Rudolf Steiner to his audience during the 'Samaritan' course in the summer of 1914. Steiner had been asked at the time for practical advice in dealing with acute war injuries, after the subject of medicine had been imposed on the small anthroposophical movement from the outside in all intensity as a result of the catastrophe of the World War. Rudolf Steiner did not, however, just teach the people gathered with him in this historic situation about various bandaging techniques (together with the Russian physician Henrietta Ginda Fritkin), but also about the inner attitude, the esoteric aspect of the therapeutic act.

The latter began, Steiner said, with the 'experience of suffering,' the inner involvement with the physical and soul hardship of the sick other person. The gospel healings often also start with Christ 'growing aware,' a far-reaching distress in the soul, a profound compassion — such as in the healing of the two blind men at Jericho:

And see, two blind men sat by the wayside. And
as they heard that Jesus was passing by, they
called out loudly: 'Lord, have pity on us, Son of
David!' The crowd rebuked them and told them
to be quiet. But they only called out even more
loudly: 'Lord, have pity on us, Son of David!'
Then Jesus stood still and called to them: 'What
do you want me to do for you?' They said, 'Lord,
that our eyes may be opened.' And Jesus felt compassion for them and touched their sight, and at
once they could see again and followed him.
(Matt.20:30–34).[9]*

The compassion of Christ leads him to come closer to
the originally distant (and hence 'crying out') sick men, to
physical contact and healing. If the power of love contained in the 'experience of suffering' and thus the partly
physical and soul identification with the needy state of the
other — feature of a future human culture — is realized,
then, according to Steiner, the power of Christ works even
today from the ego-bearing heart of the helper into the
ego-bearing heart of the sick person, and integrates both
into a unity.

Steiner's concept of the 'empathy with suffering' is in-
wardly linked with what he himself years later — in the
concept for a spiritual nurse training, jointly undertaken
with Ita Wegman — called the therapeutic 'sense of helping.' If the 'experience of suffering' turns into helping,
active love — in the sense of the overflowing, effective
love of Christ from the dimension of the organ of the heart
(or the 'I'; compare p. 121ff) — the 'sense of helping' takes
shape out of the heart sphere of the power of love:

In the heart lives
The shining brightness
Of human being's sense of helping
In the heart is active
In warming strength
The human being's power of love
So let us carry
The soul's full will
In the heart's warmth
And the heart's light
Thus we effect
Out of God's mercy
Salvation to those in need of healing.[10]*

Verse in Ita Wegman's handwriting

The second level of love we have described, the 'Christian will to heal,' can also be found in archetypal form in the healing acts in the gospels. This is particularly the case where the setting of the sick person moves towards Christ's healing power and thus creates the possibility for the substance of the healing act to be fulfilled. Thus the bearers of the stretcher with the man suffering from palsy, who in Capernaum literally took off the roof of a house to enable the sick person to come closer to Christ, possessed real *sense of helping* ('And when Jesus saw their deep trust he said to the paralysed man, "My child, you are free from the burden of your sins." ... "I say to you, stand up, take your stretcher and return to your house".' Mark 2:5, 11) The Roman soldier, too, who determinedly approached Christ to seek help for his son was acting in this spirit. His urgent *sense of helping* enabled Christ's therapeutic power to become effective and thus itself indirectly became the bearer of loving, helping power.

For the friends of a seriously ill young person Rudolf Steiner revealed the following meditation as late as February 1925, shortly before his own death:

> Loving hearts
> Warming Suns
> You traces of Christ
> In the Father's cosmos
> To you we call in our breast
> For you we search in our spirit
>   Oh, seek him out

> Radiation of the human heart
> Warmth of devoted yearning
> Homes of Christ
> In the Father's house on earth
> To you we call in our breast
> For you we search in our spirit
>   Oh, live with him.
>
> Radiating human love
> Warming sun's brightness
> Soul garments of Christ
> In the Father's human temple
> To you we call from our breast
> For you we search in our spirit
>   Oh, help him.[11]

Rudolf Steiner spoke repeatedly about the actual 'will to heal' in his medical courses in 1924. The term described by him intrinsically assumes loving experience of suffering as much as sense of helping (which both as such become part of nursing) but itself — as *will* in practice — penetrates further in professional terms towards the unconditional healing of the sick person, thus relating to the 'physician's attitude.'[12] Here the physician's 'will to heal' must connect with the 'need for healing' of the sick person, and sometimes it is the thing that stimulates it towards an effective 'will to recover.' Steiner said:

> When sick people ... simply through the individu-
> ality of the physician are brought to the point
> where they experience how the physician is
> imbued with the will to heal, there is a reflex in
> the ill person which is then penetrated by the will

Herzen, die lieben
Sonnen, die wärmen
Ihr Wegespuren Christi
In des Vaters Weltenall
Euch rufen wir aus eigner Brust
Euch suchen wir im eignen Geist
O, strebet zu ihm.

———

Menschenherzen – Strahlen
Andachtwarmes Sehnen
Ihr Heimatstätten Christi
In des Vaters Erdenhaus
Euch rufen wir aus eigner Brust
Euch suchen wir im eignen Geist
O, lebet bei ihm.

———

Strahlende Menschenliebe
Wärmender Sonnenglanz
Ihr Seelenkleider Christi
In des Vaters Menschentempel
Euch rufen wir aus eigner Brust
Euch suchen wir im eignen Geist
O, helfet in ihm.

Verse in Rudolf Steiner's handwriting (Dornach 1925)

> to recover. This collision of the will to heal and the
> will to recover plays an enormous part in
> therapy.[13]

The will to heal and the will to recover are dependent on one another, are interconnected and indicate the profound and irreplaceable significance of the therapeutic relationship.[14*] Their correspondence can once again be found in the gospels. Thus in the house of mercy at the pool of Bethesda near Jerusalem, Christ heals the paralysed man by activating his paralysed will quality ('Have you the will to become whole?' John 5:6), while the healing of the leper in Luke emphasizes the unconditional will to heal of Christ who is directly challenged to heal by the sick man:

> Once when he came to one of the towns he was
> met by a man who was completely covered in
> leprosy. When he saw Jesus he fell on his face and
> implored him: 'Lord, you can heal me clean *if you
> only will.'* Then he stretched out his hand,
> touched him and said: *'I will;* be clean!' And at
> once the leprosy left him. (Luke 5:12f, author's
> emphasis).

The will to heal is implemented healing knowledge — it is based on an act of cognition which has taken hold of the will and entirely challenges the physician at all levels of his soul.[15*] Helene von Grunelius, the 'soul' of the group of young physicians, had also received the key meditation on behalf of the group from Rudolf Steiner.[16*] In response to a corresponding question and honest personal statement by her, Rudolf Steiner expressly pointed out in his Easter course in 1924 that the initiation science of the old mysteries only made its findings available to those who worked with them on an existential and karmic

level and who had the will to turn such knowledge into
reality; finally he said to her:

> Knowledge of healing should not actually exist
> without the will to heal and you should really be
> speaking about something completely different
> today. You should not be speaking about this but
> you should really be asking: It's not been long
> since I studied medicine and now I have this over-
> whelming will to heal. I must restrain myself that
> I do not lose control of this will, which comes
> from knowledge, and start to heal people who are
> not sick.[17]

In her discussion with Rudolf Steiner on April 22, 1924
Helene von Grunelius had admitted with absolute open-
ness and honesty that although at the start of her medical
studies she had possessed a cognitive interest in the types
of illness and their treatment, she had not possessed any
actual will to heal. Steiner's partly almost sharp dispute
with her was in substance a Christologically based conflict
with Arabic medicine. 'It was not my intention to discuss
the personal characteristics of Fräulein von Grunelius, but
I wanted to characterize the kind of attitude which modern courses of necessity produce.'[18]

But the therapeutic will to heal is itself capable of further
enhancement which gives it the new quality of courage to
heal. This process occurs when the uncompromised, completely therapeutically effective will to heal also faces up
to the conflict with the opposing forces of death and in
doing so maintains its effectiveness. Rudolf Steiner told
the young physicians in January 1924:

> Such will (to heal) must never be compromised.
> Without reserve it must work therapeutically in

such a way that we can say: we will do everything, even if we are of the opinion that the
patient cannot be healed. You must suppress such
an opinion, must do everything to heal the
patient. This is meant aphoristically.'[19]

That in these words Rudolf Steiner is really referring to the
concept and the spiritual sphere of the courage to heal
became clear at most three months later when he emphasized in a meeting at Easter with practicing anthroposophical physicians

It is the worst possible thing to think of death in
respect of a sick person, be he ever so ill, if we
wish to heal him. As physicians we should virtu-
ally forbid ourselves to think of the death of the
patient as any kind of possibility. After all, the
imponderables have such a strong effect. It is an
incredibly strengthening force if you banish all
thoughts of death under all circumstances to the
last — to the very last! — and only think what
you can do to save of life forces what can be
saved. If such an attitude is developed, many
more people will be saved than if the other attitude develops which on any kind of basis fore-
casts death. We should never do that. Such things
must be properly taken into account. Then we are
entitled to have the courage to heal.[20]

In maintaining the healing intention in the conflict
with the illness-related forces of destruction, the courage
to heal — according to further explanations of Steiner —
is also enhanced, that is, it represents the will to heal
maintained in a highly dynamic borderline situation, in
that it carries spiritual knowledge of a therapeutic kind
into a potential death zone. Repeatedly — and against an

autobiographical background — Steiner, using the example of smallpox and its treatment, describes the importance of the physician courageously carrying his healing knowledge, turned will, to the patient; and that he should do so even if the latter is suffering from an infectious disease.[21]* He told the young physicians:

> If you walk into a sick room in fear, none of your therapy will help. If you enter with love, if you can ignore yourself; indeed, if you can live in love in your imaginative, inspired cognition, then you will become part of the healing process not as the fearful cognitive personality but as the loving cognitive personality.[22]

Spiritual knowledge of healing which has turned into the will to heal protects the physician in such situations not just from being infected himself, but enables the process of spiritual management of a combination of forces which the patient in his physical image suffers as disease. The courage to heal thus leads to a spiritual clash with the forces active in the progress of the illness in which the physician engages — on behalf of the patient, we might say — and which he has to face up to on an existential level within the meaning of a medicine based in Christianity. ('That means, anyone seeking their own personal happiness should not strive to embark on the path towards Raphael' Gerhard Kienle.[23]) But with that we have already touched on the next and highest sphere: therapeutic karmic resolve.

Christ, Lucifer and Ahriman:
about karmic resolve

*These two forces (Lucifer and Ahriman) are
constantly battling in the human individuality.
And the human individuality has become the scene
for the battle between Lucifer and Ahriman.*

Rudolf Steiner[24]

The construction and style of Rudolf Steiner's medical course was not 'intellectual' as such but there was a specific motif in the selected form of presentation: the spiritual scientific encouragement of the way in which the understanding of the individual physician developed. Always targeted and consistent, it was concerned with the 'independent judgment of the physician.'[25] Steiner wished to develop the therapy in methodological terms on the basis of the pathology so that it could be clearly understood and rationally founded. Also in respect of choosing possible medicines from the realms of nature, Steiner by no means endeavoured to spread his immense medical knowledge as widely as possible but, rather, to encourage his listeners to develop their own activity — they were to be *equipped* such that they could make their independent *observation* of nature. But the medicines which had already been developed were to be made *comprehensible* to the individual physicians.[26] That is why Steiner also refrained from developing medically relevant *esoteric facts*, which he might well have done, because he wished to build on the scientific basis of the physicians and to expand those ideas.[27]*

The major lecture cycle on the philosophy of Thomas Aquinas (Whitsun 1920), held in the aftermath of the first medical course (March/April 1920), provided impressive justification for such a course of action. In this, Steiner referred directly to the medical course. In doing so, he made quite clear that it was the historic task of anthroposophy to continue developing the abstract body-soul relationship in Thomas in concrete terms, to resume the battle with positivistic science — and to do so by means of the (non-intellectual) 'deepening of the life of ideas,' by a 'penetration with Christ' of the thinking.[28] To the extent that the individual succeeds by use of all his strength in breaking through the 'barrier to cognition which is the original sin of thought,' in deepening, spiritualizing and 'redeeming' his ideational capacity, the penetration of science and medicine with Christ becomes possible.[29]

This dimension of this theme of cognition in medicine, which has remained highly relevant to the present day, was outlined by Rudolf Steiner in April 1924 — in response to a corresponding question — using the example of the effectiveness of medicines as follows:

> But now let me ask you in all faith: how are the studies undertaken outside [with regard to the effectiveness of medicines]? They are undertaken quite superficially with the help of statistics, they are done in such a way that so and so many patients are given the medicine. People don't really know what is happening. The great difference between a real medicine and such a medicine is that in a real medicine you understand the process and know the effect on the human being throughout life. When you remedy something

today with some medicine you cannot know what
effect it will have in five years. But when you
understand the process completely, you do not
need any statistics. With our medicines we never
deal with statistics. You will see from the book
which is shortly to be published [*Fundamentals of
Therapy*] how whether a medicine works or not
does not depend on statistics but on the study of
individual cases. If you have a box of matches and
try a match, you do not need to burn all matches
but know that each one will burn. Similarly you
know that each process must occur in the way that
is familiar to you. It is not, therefore, about statistics, but about understanding the individual case.
... The key thing with regard to such medicines
which heal without us understanding the process
is, above all, to understand what is happening.[30]

Steiner warned urgently against the future exclusion of
the physician from the real therapeutic situation through
the health insurance companies and the enforced positivistic operation of science. He clearly saw coming a
depersonalized medicine with formalized evaluation and
treatment templates. Such a development has set in on a
sustained basis and determines the 'healing trade' more
than ever today.[31] The complete negation of any individual judgment by the physician ('to guard against any use
of judgment'[32]), the clinical study logically controlled by
'double blind' tests as the 'gold standard' and only
decisive instrument of any medicine tests, the commonly
practiced procedure to formulate 'objective' treatment
guidelines removed from the individual therapeutic situation between the patient and his physician, and thus
removed from the individual cognitive situation:

this type of thinking single-mindedly sets out to prepare the human being like a component in a giant mechanism as a useful object of society. ... The link between this impulse and the [Academy of] Gondishapur [or Arabic-Islamic medicine, author's note] is accessible to our power of judgment. Thus an impulse is revealed here which directly denies the human individual.'[33]

The style of Rudolf Steiner's medical courses should also be seen against this background and in its Christological dimensions. The deepening and spiritualization of the life of ideas, the promotion of the cognitive abilities of the treating physician, his existential entry into each specific therapy situation are then revealed to be prerequisites in the history of consciousness for a future medicine based in Christianity which respects each patient as an individual and takes account of his destiny.[34]* But for medicine today it is more than ever true that 'The human being is left out of account; karma is given a slap in the face.'[35]

'When we meet again, I will tell you how the Ahrimanic forces are intent on killing the karma of the human being dead in order to achieve their purpose.'[36] The third course by Rudolf Steiner for the group around Helene von Grunelius, which had been planned for September 1924, never happened. At the end of September of the same year Rudolf Steiner had to take to his sick bed. Thus he could no longer report how the Ahrimanic forces are intent — particularly in modern medicine — to 'kill the karma of the human being.' Karmic resolve had previously been described by Steiner as the essential prerequisite for a therapeutic attitude and for therapeutic action and we referred to invincible karmic resolve as a professional necessity for the physician.[37] The healing physician has to have an 'intimate relationship' with karma, has to treat the patient in a 'karmic sense' and be involved in his future destiny, that is, his developing karma.[38] In the medical courses, however, which were always characterized by many questions from the audience and directly related to practice, the subjects which were thus touched upon were merely hinted at in the time available. For 'The way in which karma works in human life — this question really does require to be deepened in a thorough cosmic way.'[39]

But to the extent that, according to Rudolf Steiner, Christ became the master of karma for human life in the course of the twentieth century, the associated problems play a role in the understanding of anthroposophical medicine as medicine based on Christianity.[40] Starting points for the further investigation of karmic resolve as a continuation of the will to heal, and thus of the necessary cosmic deepening — leading to the threefold figure of Christ, Lucifer and Ahriman — can be found in numerous lectures by Rudolf Steiner in which he at least partially develops the esoteric facts which are left out of consideration in the medical courses. We will consider them below, for 'if we can investigate matters with heightened cognition, we will be able to understand on a more profound level the true nature and the full significance of being ill and being healthy in human life.'[41]

Since 1909, the representation of Christ, Lucifer and Ahriman was a constant theme in Rudolf Steiner's teachings — the cognitive representation of the 'three impulses determining human evolution.'[42] In expansive excurses with subtle differences Steiner described to his listeners the intervention in evolution of those high beings, adversaries of God, with regard to the development of the human being. He illuminated the nature of their being, their power and force form. The listening anthroposophists were able to gain an advance impression of Lucifer and Ahriman — for according to Steiner the human spirit soul also encounters these divine adversary forces in its development after death in a very concrete way, indeed *walks* with them.[43] But such advance knowledge, such beginning cognition allows human beings in a certain way to protects themselves against their continuing influences. 'When we start to see him [Lucifer or Ahriman], we can protect ourselves against him.'[44*]

Steiner repeatedly emphasized the necessity of gaining knowledge about these two figures who enabled the premature individualization and autonomy of the human being in evolution, something they are now increasingly preventing, indeed destroying: 'The only thing we can say is that we are approaching free will to the extent that we succeed in mastering the influences of Lucifer and Ahriman. And we can master them only through cognition.'[45] This cognitive work results in increasing self and world knowledge and thus in an understanding of development. Lucifer and Ahriman made possible the first liberation of the human being but then led to a fixation of each person on his own human ego nature and on the mirage of the external material world; undermined the loving will as much as reflection about the essence of things; destroyed and destroy the connection of the past with the existence of the future.[46*]

> These two powers [Lucifer and Ahriman] are con-
> stantly fighting in the human individuality. And
> the human individuality has become the scene for

the battle between Lucifer and Ahriman. At the same time, the spiritual observation of physiological and anatomical processes will lead us to an understanding of how Lucifer and Ahriman are battling.[47]

In none of the medical courses are these esoteric medical facts mentioned — but in other contexts we find repeatedly a wealth of material about what Steiner said about these matters. Thus in November 1914 he discussed the spatial structure of the human body as a differentiated expression of the battles described above, and supplemented this with further information in December of the same year.[48] One year earlier, aspects of a general and individual developmental physiology against the background of Luciferic and Ahrimanic forces had been revealed by Steiner in detailed lectures, in which, among other things, the human sensory organization and the specific structure of the human life processes had been presented from a cosmic evolutionary perspective.[49]*

In the early summer of 1916, one year before the first presentation of the threefold physiology in Berlin, Steiner spoke, also in Berlin, about the polarity of blood and nerves and in this context not only characterized for the first time the nervous system as a cosmic living, but earthly dead organization (as well as the blood as an earthly dead being only capable of life in connection with the cosmic organism), but showed in essential respects that this physiological situation represented the prerequisite for Ahriman's intervention in the organ of the nervous system, whereas the blood was utilised by Lucifer. Steiner then further spoke, also for the first time, about the central motif of a threefold physiology of the human being. He said:

By having entrusted our nervous system for development to the earth, we have entrusted it to becoming dead and we have left its life up there. The life we have left up there is the same which later followed in the being of Christ. The life of our nerves, which we do not carry in us, which we have not been able to carry in us from the start of our existence on earth, followed in the being of Christ. And what was it, that it had to grasp in earth existence? It had to grasp the blood! That is the reason for the constant reference to the mystery of the blood. What is divided in us because the nervous system lost its cosmic life and the blood gained cosmic life, because life turned into death and death turned into life, that established a new connection through the element which does not live in our earthly nervous system descending from the cosmos, becoming human being, entering the blood; and the blood combined with the earth. ... And we, as human beings, can balance the polarity between our nervous system and our blood system through our participation in the mystery of Christ.[50]

The spiritual background (and the esoteric facts) of polarity and balance (or mediation) in the physiology of the human being was developed by Steiner in the context of the evolving trinity of Christ, Lucifer and Ahriman in 1916 and further elaborated in the following years.[51] In a corresponding Dornach lecture in January 1922, in which Steiner spoke about the link between the Luciferic blood forces and the development of temperature and fever in humans, contrasting this with the Ahrimanic character of the nervous sclerotic forces, he said towards the end of his account:

The study of human health and pathology will only be put on a healthy footing when these polarities in the physical human being are seen everywhere. We will then know, for example, that when the second dentition appears in human beings at around the age of seven, the Ahrimanic forces become active in relation to the head aspects; that when the human being's physical nature develops towards the warmth aspects on reaching sexual maturity, the Luciferic forces are at work, and that in his rhythmical nature the human being constantly swings, also in a physical respect, between Luciferic and Ahrimanic nature. Only when we learn to speak without superstition but with scientific precision about the Luciferic and Ahrimanic element in human nature in the same way that today we speak without superstition, without mystification of positive and negative magnetism, will we be in a position to gain knowledge of the human being which is the equal of the abstract knowledge of inorganic nature which we have achieved in the course of recent centuries.[52]

In terms of the history of culture and of consciousness, but also medically and physiologically, the destructive influence of Ahrimanic forces dominates on a sustained basis in our time. According to Rudolf Steiner, Ahriman takes possession of the human being on the way to incarnation by force, resulting in premature incarnation, takes hold 'of human thinking with his own thinking with powerful haste, with powerful energy. He hooks into the brain, we might say. Ahriman seeks to tie human beings more and more to the earth.'[53] This creates the depersonalized, deindividualized intelligence of human beings, in other words, the anti-Michaelic separation of the thinking from the feeling will. Ahrimanic intelligence dominates science as much as it occupies — with the help of destructive beings — technology, industry and commerce, creating in the end (after destruction of the realms of nature) a world which is a fully materialized mechanism, a 'Saturn of machines': 'We are only witnessing the beginning of such activity .... It will grow stronger and stronger, more and more radical.'[54]

As Rudolf Steiner described in a lecture in Vienna at Whitsun 1922 ('Anthroposophy as striving to penetrate the world with Christianity'), Ahriman — preparing his real incarnation in the third millennium — is increasingly also instrumentalizing the elemental beings in nature for his purposes.[55] 'This is what is today hanging in the spiritual world as an overwhelming decision: to create an alliance between the Ahrimanic forces and the forces of nature.'[56] Thus a world is progressively being created — not least with the help of a science subject to Ahriman — in which there is no longer any room for biographical developmental processes, which negates the individual, which extinguishes the human individuality. As we have already quoted, Rudolf Steiner told the young physicians: 'When we meet again, I will tell you how the Ahrimanic forces are intent on killing the karma of the human being dead in order to achieve their purpose.'[57]

As early as 1910, Steiner had said in Hamburg:
> What we acquire on earth as the healthy power of
> judgment is something of which Ahriman is terri-
> bly afraid. Nothing is basically as abhorrent to
> him as what we achieve through the healthy train-

ing of our ego-consciousness. ... So the more we
endeavour to develop what we can acquire as
healthy judgment in life between birth and death,
the more we work in opposition to Ahriman.[58]

In terms of the establishment of a medicine based on
Christianity this means — wholly in the sense described
above with regard to the medical courses — that such a
medicine in the present time requires the unconditional
enhancement and thus spiritualization of the forces of
thinking of the individual. From the beginning, Steiner
demanded of anthroposophical doctors that they should
come to grips with the scientific system of university medicine in order to wrest from this system — with the help of
a careful differentiation between fruitful empirical research
results and erroneous theoretical premises of methodological materialism — its inherent (but Ahrimanically dis-
torted) truth content. But whereas the physicians around
Rudolf Steiner were not able to take on this Christian and
Aristotelian scientific task,[59*] a physician like Gerhard
Kienle faced up to it after the Second World War at an existential level.[60] In Kienle's last Dornach lecture in September 1981 he put it like this:

What was the actual significance of Alexander
the Great so that Rudolf Steiner referred to
'Alexandrism'? Despite his youth, he possessed
a quite extraordinary drive and resolution and
developed sweeping perspectives. It had been his
fortunate destiny to have been taught by one of
the greatest minds in Greece, to have immediately
picked up and implemented the brilliant strategic
planning of his father after his death despite the
deep rift between them, and to have left no
karmic situation out of account and unused with

regard to the overall objective. Greece was the intellectual centre of the time and Greece had to vanquish Persia if it was to maintain its position. Alexander realized that an impetuous will which subjects itself to mental discipline can conquer the problems of the world. *Today* the point at issue is that world problems should be understood as *conflicts about truth and ideas* and that the same penetrating resolution which Alexander realized on the physical level is brought to bear in the spiritual conflict. Such spiritual willingness to engage in combat which only asks after truth and not after the security of existence would be Alexandrism. But it must combine with Aristotelianism. At the same time Rudolf Steiner always spoke of the necessity of returning to Aristotel's ten categories for reading in the book of nature. What does this mean? It means nothing other than in the scientific field dealing with basic questions in every respect. The battle front in spiritual conflict lies in the field of the so-called axiomatic. This includes the concept of matter in the natural sciences. Not for nothing did Rudolf Steiner concern himself with the concept of the atom from the beginning. Aristotelianism and Alexandrism working together can defeat the demons of Bacon.[61]

Together with working with empirical science in this way and engaging with its ideas, Steiner in a further step called for the creation of an original Christian natural science with an anthroposophical orientation, also as the foundation for a Christianized medicine. Here he made clear in the Vienna lecture of Whitsun 1922, already cited, that such a natural science penetrated by Christianity had to be connected with the elemental beings to counter by Christian means the threatening alliance between Ahriman and the spirits of nature. This motif could already be cautiously heard in the Whitsun lectures about Thomas Aquinas from 1920. A spiritual natural science with an orientation towards spiritual science led to knowledge of spiritual beings, Steiner said at the time.[62]

During Steiner's lifetime, Lili Kolisko quite obviously worked wholly in the spirit of such intentions. Although not directly discussed by Steiner in this way, the spiritual background of her scientific work appears to be penetrated with Christianity in the sense referred to and to be connected with the elemental beings. As early as their first meeting, Steiner acknowledged her pronounced spiritual perception in a deepened scientific sense ('You can see the ether'[63]), and subsequently repeatedly discussed not only her work — despite negative criticism from among the anthroposophical physicians — in a very positive way but also included her in the medical lectures and the curative education course, allowed her to takes notes in the class lessons and speak about them in Stuttgart. In order, finally, to bring Lili Kolisko's scientific work once more urgently to the attention of the members, he let her lecture in detail at the Goetheanum on December 31, 1923, the anniversary of the fire. He himself spoke the mantra of the Foundation Stone verse:

> Light divine,
> Sun of Christ
> The elemental spirits hear it
> in East, West, North, South
> May human beings hear it.[64]

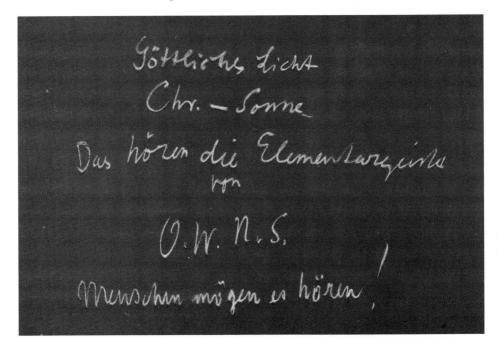

Rudolf Steiner's verse as he wrote it on the blackboard in 1923

'If we can investigate matters with heightened cognition, we will be able to understand on a more profound
level the true nature and the full significance of being ill
and being healthy in human life.'[65] In at least three major
lectures and courses Rudolf Steiner spoke about therapeutic and karmic issues against the background of the trinity
of Christ, Lucifer and Ahriman and in connection with
concrete clinical pictures — and indirectly about 'karmic
resolve.' He did so in greatest detail in the early Hamburg
course about 'Manifestations of karma' (May 1910), then
on November 16, 1917 in St Gallen ('I have spoken here
today as I have because — how should I put this? — that
is what the genius loci demanded of me'), and finally in an
intense, indeed, dramatic way exactly five years later

(November 16, 1922) in London, the home city of Edith Maryon, shortly before the Dornach fire and Edith Maryon's illness.[66]

One fundamental aspect of 'karmic resolve,' as Rudolf Steiner called it, was discussed as early as the Vienna lecture which has already been quoted, 'Anthroposophy as striving to penetrate the world with Christianity.' Steiner spoke about his spiritual scientific research into rickets ('But I observed ...') and emphasized that the soul of the incarnating child has a karmic affinity with the specific conditions of its environment in early childhood, but therefore also to those circumstances which could promote or enable rickets to occur:

> Down to the individual details, the sympathies of
> the soul encompass that which draws the children
> to a life on earth, down to the individual details
> the souls encompass that which draws them to the
> life they must live, perhaps in a room that faces
> north or a room that faces south. A soul may want
> to develop in the dark under certain circum-
> stances. We must not say that we should only look
> out for the one factor, whether there is sufficient
> light or air, but we must look to the soul and spirit
> which was longing for such an environment. ...
> That is why we must ask ourselves: should we
> only attempt to heal what we perceive as rickets in
> accordance with the physical conditions which we
> learn about through physical cognition? We should
> not, but must tell ourselves: if we managed to take
> the medicine such that the person simply recov-
> ered physically, he would have to push down into
> the deepest depths of his soul life those things
> which lie in his destiny and which caused him to

long for a world not filled with light. And only if we succeed in also taking account of those things which have gone into the subconscious, if we enable the person to bring to consciousness what he has to do, only if we look at the whole person as body, soul and spirit, can we establish a comprehensive science, including medicine.[67]

Any therapeutic intervention influences the destiny of the patient, but it is helpful and healing *in a karmic sense* only if reversing the physical course of the illness is combined with more comprehensive assistance in overcoming the actual background to the illness. Similarly Steiner had emphasized twelve years earlier in the Hamburg karma lectures — using the example of the smallpox infection (see above, p 57f) — that it was the task of the therapist, that is, the physician physically getting rid of the disease, to create a 'spiritual counterpart' to the organic problem: 'For if we do nothing further, we have only done half our work, if any at all.'[68] And to this extent to help the patient to convert the dynamic of forces which have taken a physical form back into their original spiritual and soul process in order then to achieve change at that level.

Thus karmic resolve in the first instance means that the physician does not just help on a physical level, but also implements the absolutely essential spiritual counterpart to the organic illness and is thus prepared down to the cognitive process to expose himself selflessly to the actual causative forces of the disease. Without such a spiritual confrontation, effective methods of healing cannot be found.[69]* As Gerhard Kienle puts it:

When the physician crosses the threshold ... he must really take on the inner burden of the problem contained in the destiny of the patient and pass through the drama of overcoming it himself, because beyond the threshold we cannot remain uncommitted. This means that the person who crosses the threshold in this way takes on karmic burdens which are comparable to constantly being affected by new misfortunes. This should only take place in the soul and spirit and not in external destiny — which cannot always be avoided — but that does not make the drama of overcoming misfortune any less. ... To illustrate this with an image: if a ship has been shipwrecked and rescuers go out in a lifeboat to save those who are shipwrecked, they are exposed to the same storms and forces of nature as the shipwrecked people, except that the lifeboat men do not expose themselves recklessly but with the motive of rendering assistance to those in trouble.[70]

The 'elemental forces' which the treating physician has to face on a spiritual level are in essence Lucifer and Ahriman. In 1910, Rudolf Steiner described for the first time, and in exceptional detail, how the sick person in dealing with the process of his disease on an organic level is able to liberate himself from a one-sided orientation towards Ahriman or Lucifer in his last incarnation.[71]*

The process of coping with the disease creates an absolutely necessary and deeply meaningful liberation from the anti-divine forces — even if the illness ends in death.[72]* If the physical treatment by the physician combats nothing other than the process of organic disease — or if, indeed, the treatment prevents the process altogether — the task in relation to destiny is merely pushed into deeper layers of the soul life and obviously made more difficult. Any therapeutic intervention is therefore only truly healing from the perspective of spiritual science if the physician himself — practicing a radical karmic resolve — cognitively opposes the occurrence of the Luciferic and Ahrimanic powers in the patient and is able to show and accompany the patient in other ways of prevailing. Such a medical and therapeutic attitude can quite clearly begin to be experienced in its spiritual undertaking by the patient: 'Patients were able to experience the devoted sacrificial willingness [of Dr Helene von Grunelius] to take on the illness of her fellow human beings in order to overcome it.'[73]

The real drama contained in this spiritual process — the wholly existential dimension of which was possessed not least by Rudolf Steiner's own cognitive work in this field (as exemplary Christian cognitive medicine),[74*] — was developed with brilliant intensity in the London lecture of November 16, 1922 mentioned above. In it Steiner not only described Lucifer's and Ahriman's battle against one another in the human being as well as their specific conflict with the planetary spirits, but he also described the diseases as the *last defence* of human beings against the (almost) victorious adversary powers. In certain situations only such (somatic and psychiatric) illnesses enabled the human being to be maintained — leading, finally, to defeat for Lucifer and Ahriman: 'One has the strongest impression of Ahriman's and Lucifer's disappointment when one visits hospitals and sickbeds or mental asylums.'[75] Speaking about his own spiritual scientific observations in this dynamic force field, Steiner said at the end of the London lecture:

> When we cross the threshold, consciously look
> into the spiritual world and this terrible battle,

when we observe this confusing game for the human being behind nature and below it, then in the present time we will look in vain for these messengers of the gods who for instance presented the ancient mystery physicians with the rod of mercury and similar symbols to do with healing. It is difficult to cope with this terrible battle ... And it is truly the case that when you cross the threshold you are placed in the midst of this terrible battle ... And the battle takes place beyond the threshold in a terrible way, so that the Sun first becomes very fiery and the darkens until at the end it appears like a black disc.

This was not what is was like for the initiates. They saw through the disc turned black. And precisely out of this disc turned black they encountered the divine messengers of the Father who in ancient times were the carriers of medical knowledge.

We modern people cross the threshold and are faced with this terrible battle. The Sun turns red, the Sun turns black, but it remains a black disc. And we are turned back and have to search on earth itself in order to find our way in this terrible battle.

Here we are referred to Christ, who stands there as the spiritual being which has united itself with the earth through the mystery of Golgotha and tells us: Do not despair that the sun has turned black; it has turned black because I, the Sun god, am no longer there but have descended to earth and united with it. ...

And it is Christ who indicates the resources in

the human being to reconcile the upper [Luciferic] with lower [Ahirmanic] forces ... And particularly as human beings we are then given guidelines both for healing illness and for an understanding of all the other evils, which always disappoints Lucifer and Ahriman. And we reach a stage through the power of Christ and the power of the Mystery of Golgotha to be able to speak what I would call the wonderful words: You creatures of Ahriman and Lucifer, your are disappointed by evils which have to arise on earth through you in that you achieve your victories, your partial victories. These disappointments of yours will keep coming back because you will always continue ... to produce sick and obsessed people. And so you will rush from delirious joy to saddest disappointment.

But human beings on earth, if they find the correct relationship to Christ, have been given the instrument to hand not to despair in such a moment where they experience the despair of higher beings than themselves; higher beings, but higher beings who are embarked on a different path to those divine beings of whom human beings are a part and to whom they should remain loyal in the further course of earth development. The focus of these divine beings is the being of Christ which a long time ago spoke to the ancient initiates through the disc of the Sun and who speaks to us again from earth with the help of the Sun. So when we speak of Christ today we speak of the one who can accompany us on earth as the guide who guides us away from the terrible struggle of the Ahrimanic and Luciferic forces

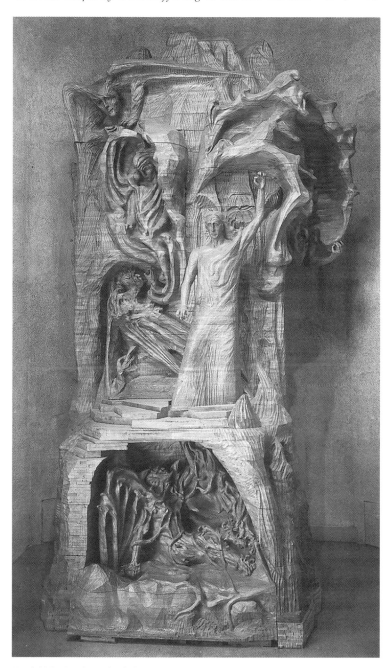

Rudolf Steiner's and Edith Maryon's sculpture (Dornach, 1925)

among one another and against the higher and lower divine worlds.[76]

In the sculptural group created by Rudolf Steiner together with Edith Maryon, karmic resolve understood in this way was given shape in a world historical context. In it Christ the Saviour overcomes the adversary forces with the purest gesture of compassion. The radiating creative love of the 'master of karma' which extends even to the fallen adversary forces cannot be born by Lucifer and Ahriman, leading to their retreat and self-destruction. The gospels in turn report how Christ comes to terms with Lucifer and Ahriman in the situations when he is subject to temptation, how he takes the destiny of illness of those in need spiritually on himself and thus cosmically redeems it ('But Jesus only bent down and wrote with his finger in the earth' that is, on his own 'I'; John 8:6), thus healing the sick people physically while at the same time guiding each of them towards their own developmental goal. This process of culmination of therapeutic karmic resolve is illustrated by Rudolf Frieling in his exposition of the central healing of the blind man in the Gospel of St John (compare pp. 32ff), the healing treatment which leads to a real experience of Christ — 'I am the good shepherd, and know my sheep, and am known of mine' — through a deeper understanding of the individual.[77]

Christian medicine had its beginnings in the healing acts of Christ. The path of Luke for training a therapeutic *attitude,* initiated by Rudolf Steiner in the twentieth century, leads back to that source which is the constant and continuing paradigm for a new medicine.

3. The Healing Medicine

Communion and Medicine

> *Writing history means giving dates their physiognomy.*
>
> Walter Benjamin.[1]

The year 1922 was when the Christian Community was founded. In 1923 Rudolf Steiner began his closer collaboration with Ita Wegman for the creation of a new mystery medicine. But 1922 was also the year in which the first volume of the collected scientific writings of the physician Theophrastus von Hohenheim, called Paracelsus, was published. In the following year, the complete edition (still not concluded) of his theological manuscripts was started.

The whole of the work of the early sixteenth-century hermit physician, which now began to appear, was focused on medicine, on healing substance and healing. His theological writings, published from 1923 onwards, which centred on the sacrament of communion, were also for the sick and people in need. Rudolf Steiner's fundamental book with Ita Wegman, work on which began in

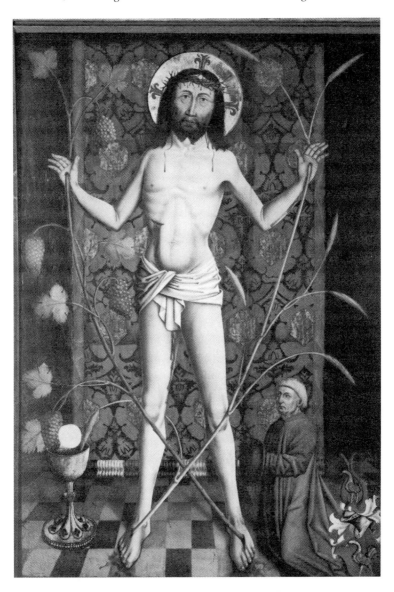

Portrayal of Christ from school of Friedrich Herlin (Nördlingen, 1469)

1923, in turn built on the spiritual scientific description of human physical substance and methodologically set out the path to healing substance. And the Christian Community, founded in 1922 with Steiner's assistance, sees its spiritual focus in the celebration of the mass and thus the transubstantiation.[2*]

Only five days had passed since Friedrich Rittelmeyer had celebrated the first complete Act of Consecration of Man when Rudolf Steiner told his listeners in Dornach on September 21, 1922 almost out of the blue:

> Just imagine, a personality lived in Paracelsus for whom religion applied so widely that it included medicine. In Paracelsus there lived a concept of religion which enabled him to keep hold of the spiritual in such a way that one can penetrate oneself with it right into the illness, so that the physician is the person who carries out the will of God on earth with regard to sick people. For him medical service was religious service. And that is something which is very necessary today: not just to talk eternally about the eternal, but to carry the eternal into all of life and to bring it to life and activate it in all living things.[3]

And eight days later, on Michaelmas Day 1922, he said:

> As a physician, Paracelsus wanted to be a religious and pious person. The individual medical act, the therapeutic act, was to be a religious act. For him his actions with the patient were a unification of the external physical human act with religious observance. Fundamentally he still saw healing as a religious act. And it was his ideal to turn it into a religious act.[4]

The following account investigates the path of healing
substance which was indicated by both Paracelsus and
Rudolf Steiner in medical and theological respects. Even if
the substance of a medicine is essentially different from
that of communion — which was stressed and shown by
Paracelsus *and* Rudolf Steiner with great emphasis — it
should not be forgotten that humankind over many centuries experienced the inner relationship of both. For long
periods the 'daily bread,' the daily nourishment of the
human being, was understood in a healing sense; the Old
High German word *nerjan* or *neren* and the Middle High
German *nerigen* (modern German *nähren,* to nourish)
according to Grimms *Deutsches Wörterbuch* contained the
meaning of 'keeping alive,' 'making healthy,' 'healing';
and the word *Genesung* (recovery), still in use today, has
the verb *neren* in its root. Sanctification, in turn, has
implied since ancient times a healing of the human being
and was originally unthinkable without it; but this means
that it also always has an aspect closely connected with
the body and medicine. Thus we can read about the *Grail*
in Wolfram von Eschenbach that its power not only physically nourished the whole of the Grail company *(si lebent
von einem steine* — they lived from a stone) but the fatally
sick King Anfortas was kept alive through it alone. All this
can be done by the 'Stone' (as revealed by Trevrizent)
because a brilliantly white dove once a year, on Good
Friday, laid on it a small white wafer which brings the
power of the grail.[5]

In the gospels, Christ already transforms earth substance while he is still alive and gives it healing proper-
ties. Sight is restored to the man born blind through the
'paste' of the earth which Christ prepares for him, using
his own saliva, and places on his eyes (John 9:6). And in

the synagogue at Capernaum the words were heard early on:

> I AM the life-giving bread which descends from heaven. Whoever eats of this bread will live through all cycles of time. And the bread which I shall give — that is my earthly body which I shall offer up for the life of the world. ... Whoever eats my body and drinks my blood has life beyond the cycles of time, and I give him the power of resurrection at the end of time. For my flesh is the true sustenance, and my blood is the true draught. Whoever truly eats my flesh and drinks my blood remains in me and I in him. (John 6:51, 54–56).

Paracelsus

> *How can I not appear strange to him who has never*
> *walked in the sun?*
>
> Paracelsus[6]

Throughout his life, the physician Paracelsus remained an isolated, itinerant outsider, envied for his therapeutic success, hated or ridiculed for his appearance and ideas. His countless writings on medicine, natural science and theology — notes created while travelling and maintaining the characteristics of the spoken word — were mostly published after his death and not always then. The edition of his theological works, started by Wilhelm Matthiessen in 1923, still has not reached beyond volume seven of twelve after almost eight decades of editing. The collection of his writings on the communion, the arrival of which as Volume 10 has been announced for a long time, still lies in the far distant future.[7*] Despite his rediscovery at the end of the nineteenth century by the medical historian Karl Sudhoff, a peculiar, impeding fate still hangs over the revolutionary spiritual work of the hermit physician. Already during Paracelsus' lifetime, he fought against it and railed against his enemies. But then the sentence follows: 'How can I not appear strange to him who has not walked in the sun?'

Paracelsus' main medical concern was the healing of the sick. But according to Gunhild Pörksen[8] all his writings are devoted to that fundamental phenomenon of medicine, *human development*. Here is thoughts on physical development through the nutritional process as well as his theological ideas on the development of the 'eternal body' through the sacrament take central place.

With regard to the human nutritional processes, Paracelsus repeatedly emphasized that they implied the complete transformation and ingestions into the body of non-human nourishment. But transformation here means in the first instance the 'separation' of the 'essence' of the nutritional substance of benefit to human beings from the always present and potentially fatal poison. Because every substance which is alien to the organism is harmful as such although it may be fully developed in itself. The organ for such necessary 'separation' is the stomach, a 'great artist' and 'alchemist' as Paracelsus described it

> This is the Alchemist, described as such with reason, because he uses the art of alchemy. He separates the bad from the good, transforms the good into a tincture, he administers to the body to give it life, he creates order in nature's subject, he administers it such that it becomes flesh and blood. This alchemist lives in the stomach which is an instrument in which he cooks and works.[9]

The final objective of the physical process of nourishment is the real internalization of alien matter, that is, the transformation of substance into 'flesh and blood' of the human being. Such transformation of matter 'in us or to us' is clearly a very far-reaching process in the sense that Paracelsus understood it.[10] He also described it as destructive fire or rotting process, in other words a real transition through death which must precede the 'other birth' in the sense of a new formation of substance by the organism itself.[11]

A fundamentally similar process is asserted by

Paracelsus for the 'alchemical' preparation of medicines, indeed he repeatedly compared the process of the digestion and formation of nourishment with the pharmacopoeic transformation of substance prescribed by the physician. This is absolutely necessary since according to Paracelsus no untransformed earth substance can be regarded as medicine:

> Because nature is so subtle and sharp in its things
> that it cannot be used without great skill because
> it reveals nothing which is complete in its type
> but must be completed by human beings. Such
> completion is called alchemy. Because the baker in
> baking bread, the vintner in making wine, the
> weaver in making cloth, is an alchemist. The same
> person who brings what in nature grows for the
> benefit of human beings to the place where it was
> ordered by nature is an alchemist.[12]

In this context the pharmacopoeic transformation process is only on the correct path, according to Paracelsus, if it finally results in the renewed opening of the created substance to the formative cosmic forces. It is these (described by Paracelsus as *arcanum)* which in the final instance make medicine effective:

> If it is now to come about that your medicine be
> as complete as the summer brings its fruits, then
> know that summer does it through the stars and
> not without them. So to the extent that the stars
> do it, know here also that the preparation must be
> such that it is subject to the stars because they are
> the ones that complete the work of the physician.[13]

But this process which prepares earthly substances primarily in the stars, is by nature also a destructive process.

Only the 'fracture' of the substances, that is, the cancellation of their own physical laws, 'aerates' them and allows the cosmic influences to work:

> Such arcanum is chaos and the stars can guide it
> like a feather is guided by the wind. ... Hence
> know this alone, that it is the arcana which are
> virtues and powers, which are volatilia or volatile,
> and have no corpora, and are chaos and are
> clarum, that is bright, and are lucent and are in
> the power of the stars.[14]

On this basis the physician preparing his medicines must in the first instance know — just like the great 'separator' of the stomach — the constitution of natural things in order to be able to 'fracture' them properly and make them accessible to higher influences: 'If he does not know these things — how nature is composed — how can he then dissolve them? Know, that you must dissolve! Go back the way! All the works done by nature, from one stage to the next, you must undo again.'[15] If the natural substances encounter human beings in untransformed forms of existence, then according to Paracelsus they are in a state of 'intermediate life' between original *prima materia* and possible *ultima materia,* and thus in a developed state of latency which requires further development. In this intermediate state of latency the possible forces of earth substance are not revealed and do not become effective since they require the cosmic influence for that. Untransformed earth substance by itself is therefore never healing substance and hides its corresponding qualities:

> [So] it is like someone who sees a tree in winter,
> does not know what it is and what it contains
> until the summer comes and the shoots, blossoms,
> fruit and whatever else it contains begin to open.

> In the same way the virtue in things lies hidden to
> human beings unless human beings become
> aware of it through the alchemist like through
> summer because otherwise it is impossible for
> human beings to recognize it.[16]

If this description of the preparation of medicines is
applied back to the nutritional process — the first 'fractur-
ing' stage which Paracelsus described almost exclusively
in the account quoted above — we might ask whether
Paracelsus understood the 'new birth' of the body's own
substances also as a cosmic process, albeit taking place
within the human being. That this might be so is made
clear by a longer text passage in *Volumen Paramirum* in
which Paracelsus says that the human body contains an
autonomous structure of organs, comparable to the planetary heavens and standing in relation to them, which as
such did *not* required earth substances:

> Just as the heavens with their firmament, constel-
> lations and nothing excluded are free unto them-
> selves, so the human being is constituted
> completely unto himself. Just like the firmament
> in the heavens is unto itself and is governed by no
> creature, so the firmament in the human being,
> that is in him, is subject to no other creatures. But
> it is alone a mighty free firmament without any
> ties. So observe two creations: heaven and earth
> the one, the human being the other.[17]

Here it is specifically the seven main organs of the body,
related to the cosmic planets 'in spirit but not in substance,'[18] which do not require any nourishment in the
actual sense and which, on the contrary, support life
within the organism in their respective spheres of activity. The physical nutritional substances merely have a

stimulating sustaining significance for the remaining *corpus* of the body (which Paracelsus distinguishes from the bodily firmament like earth from heaven). Having emphasized the autonomy of the body in near absolute terms (at least as far as the main organs are concerned), he wrote:

> So you should understand that the human being also is bound in that he must take nourishment from outside; this same nourishment serves the corpus alone like manure serves the fields. It does not produce any fruit in it, does not increase the seeds in it; it does no more than sustain it in its substance and make it lusty like manure does the fields, otherwise it is of no use. Food is as much use to human beings as if it were manure.[19]

The text seems to say here that Paracelsus wished to clarify that the significance of nutrition cannot be equated with a direct enhancement of substance — something which appears excluded in principle already in the introductory explanations — but that it merely stimulates what happens quasi autonomously in the organism following the cosmic example. If we include a further text passage from this section ('Of consumption' from the text *Elf Tractat),* then at least a part of the human body tends towards direct *cosmic* dependence in terms of its substantial composition rather than primary earthly dependence. Because it says very clearly there: 'The limb which has its nourishment from heaven withdrawn, will wither.'[20]

> It is an error when people say that the limbs, the body, etc. must have nourishment; but as to the question why they must have nourishment and

for what purpose, their wisdom comes to an end.
They have not understood what nourishment is in
the human being, what it turns into and who
makes it thus. ... What is nourishment? It is not to
feed or to fill but *to give form*.[21]

Whereas the human physical substance clearly forms in
the organism in accordance with its own laws, as we have
seen from the statements quoted above, and this process is
at most stimulated and maintained by physical nourishment, Paracelsus expressly emphasizes in his later work
Opus Paramirum that 'form is given' through the internalized foodstuffs: 'There is food in everything for the sake of
form.'[22] In *this* respect, Paracelsus says, the nutritional
process is directly necessary for life and is life sustaining.
Human beings require it constantly because their 'form,'
their 'image' (clearly understood by Paracelsus as the
shape of the body and organs) is continuously destroyed
through a decomposing force resident in the human
being:

> For a being resides in us which is like fire; that
> same being gnaws away at our form and image. If
> we did not add anything and did not increase the
> form of our body, then a person would die and his
> image would be abandoned. ... Therefore know
> that all things which live feel hunger and thirst
> because of the wasting away of their form and its
> preservation so that through hunger and thirst
> they build up their image again.[23]

In this sense the taking of nourishment is like a constant
struggle against the death intrinsic to human beings,
which they suffer as 'consumption of the form': 'That self
same death must be held at bay by the human being
through what nourishment does and is able to do.'[24] But

this leads to the conclusion: 'He who fails to eat fails to grow, he who fails to eat fails to stay. ... Because health needs to be maintained in continued existence like illness.'[25]

The internalized formative shapes (or formative potentials or, indeed, formative forces) internalized by means of nutrition contain the 'image' of the human being. He himself is not regenerated in terms of his substance but in terms of his formative processes by his non-human environment. But this entails in the final instance a process of constant development towards *becoming human* of the nature which is internalized by the human being and transformed into himself:

> That is why we eat our fingers, our body, blood, flesh, feet, brain, heart, etc.; that is, each bite we take contains within it all our limbs, everything which human beings conceive of and contain within themselves.[26]
>
> In the light of nature it becomes apparent that all things are not what we take them for. Because the essence of things is hidden from our eyes. Thus everything we eat and drink contains our flesh and blood, but we do not see it. That is why we should not believe what we see. Thus we consider wheat to be flour and it is flesh and blood. Ox may be meat but clearly not human flesh. And the same is true of vegetables and all other things — they are 'human flesh in mysterio.' ... All external things are nothing other than the body of the human being.[27]
>
> Bread is blood, but who sees it?[28]

Here it should be taken into account with regard to the overall understanding of this continuous process of *becom-*

ing human that for Paracelsus the human being was the culmination of all natural creatures and that he understood them as evolutionary fragments of that form which has its holistic objective and image in the human being. Hence he was able to say: '... All creatures are letters and books describing the origin of the human being; the creatures are letters in which can be read who human beings are.'[29] Against this evolutionary background the formative potentials of the natural environment ingested by the human being are by no means primarily earth forces; on the contrary, it may be assumed that these formative forces are of cosmic origin and have merely found a temporary shape in the physical creatures before being liberated, as we might say, by human beings, internalized, enhanced and fulfilled: 'Because heaven is the human being and the human being is heaven, and all human beings are heaven and heaven is only a human being...'[30]

The body which human beings continuously build for themselves through internalizing the natural formative processes as described, was called by Paracelsus in his medical writings the 'body of mercy' and he differentiates it from the continuously consumed 'body of justice' which comes from the parents and forms the 'beginning of our human development.' Here he says in detail:

> Because justly we have a body from our father
> and mother; but that the latter should not die and
> disappear we receive ... through mercy, through
> appeal to God, in asking give us this day our
> daily bread, which is to say: Give us this day our
> daily body. For the body from our mother
> approaches the hour of its death. That is why we
> ask for our daily [bread]; the same is the daily

[bread] which gives us our body. ... That is to say, we are appointed in both bodies, in the one we have been given from our father and mother and the one we are given through our food.[31]

The appeal for our daily bread in the Lord's Prayer means in this context also, according to Paracelsus, the concern that the nourishment should be 'pure' and thus ingestible by human beings — for: 'the more like the bread, the healthier the body.'[32]

> If we are unable to grasp in the light of nature how fishes, cabbage etc. are flesh in potential and become our flesh, how mush less can we grasp what Christ gives us in bread and wine. ... Hence in nature we must follow the command of God and eat and drink if we want to preserve our physical body. God may or may not have given us understanding how cabbage turns to flesh in us. But our understanding of the body and blood of Christ is much less than even that.[33]

Thus wrote Paracelsus in his text on the Lord's Supper, which he also called Christ's Supper. The transformation of substance in the sacrament as such is inaccessible to the normal senses and ordinary human reason according to Paracelsus; nevertheless, he also holds the view that an approach to the overall context of this central Christian mystery is indeed possible through a deeper observation of nutrition. Because to the extent that in the sense set out above 'all external things ... are none other than the human body,' no one should 'wonder' how bread and wine can be designated the body and blood of Christ:

> Because, as stated, each food and each drink is our body and blood, and the human being could say of

each food and each drink: that is my body and
blood, my bone marrow etc. This is clearly no lie
because this is what can be shown to exist in nature
although our eyes do not see it. ... Cannot Christ,
who was a human being, thus speak and point to
bread and wine as body and blood and say, that is
he? Because he had flesh and blood, also a human
body like other human beings. Observe the following example: Let us assume I had enough daily
food and drink for my nutrition and needs and in
weight for my flesh and blood. Now a thirsty or
hungry person came to me and I gave him, before I
ate, half of my daily need — could I not say: he is
eating my body and drinking my blood, because I
am giving him part of my substance, of my inner
body? ... It is love which gives to one's neighbour if
someone gives of his body.[34]

The connections thus set out are explained by Paracelsus
also using a passage from the Gospel of St Mark, in which
Christ highlights the modest gift of a totally impoverished
widow in the Temple at Jerusalem ('this poor widow has
given more than all the others who have put something
into the collection box. They all gave out of their abundance; but she, although she is in need, has given everything she had, all she had left for her living' Mark 12:43f)
— on which Paracelsus comments: 'She gave a part of the
body.' At the end of these remarks, he wrote:

Is it not so, that from these or similar reports the
simple ordinary man is better able to understand
the communion of Christ, namely that we are talking about his body, even if it may not be sufficiently
clear to our external eyes and natural reason?[35]

In his text on the Lord's Supper, the central concern of the physician Paracelsus was Christ's *body.* He rejected any symbolic or metaphorical re-interpretation of the transformation of substance in the sacraments as vehemently as the theological debate which was taking place at the time. According to Paracelsus the Christian mystery should not be dissected in debate but one should learn to understand and comprehend it in 'naivety.' But, specifically, one should not 'deprive of body' what 'Christ has given body.'[36] Christ's incarnation at the turning point in time, and thus the event when the divine Son really became human (in Paracelsus' search for the appropriate formulation he took on 'spiritual flesh or spirit flesh'[37]), was for the hermit physician the event in world history against the background of which the gospels and thus also the communion had to be seen. ('Because Christ did not endow anything non-physical and was not a spirit, but a human being, the communion must be understood physically.'[38])

Christ becoming human in its continuing effect (in great extension of the temple alms) gives the human being a sacred body, a body which is now eternal and which renews the old, mortal body of Adam from the Father God while at the same time creating an alliance with the human soul (they are 'one thing'[39]). It thus cancels out human 'original sin' which caused the rift in the old body-soul relationship (leading to the mortality of the Father body). According to Paracelsus' repeated descriptions, the new Christ body has the shape of the old Adam body and is invisibly hidden within it. It is spiritual but at the same time substantial and therefore requires nourishment which is fulfilled in sacred communion: 'Look at Christ who ate fish and honey after his resurrection although he was now immortal. But it was spiritually digested and did not leave the body again. With the help of such a "digestion" we also eat physically and process it spiritually.'[40] 'We eat ourselves into eternal life.'[41]

The nourishment of the sacrament is preserved in the eternal body of the human being — Paracelsus says — and goes to the human *heart* where it remains and grows.[42] Against such a background, communion must be seen as a healing process for the whole of humankind and thus includes a resurrection event which according to Paracelsus forms the beginning of the realm of God upon earth. But its real origin lies in Golgotha. The spilling of the blood of Christ and its uniting with the earth means, according to Paracelsus, in this sense precisely the start of redemption just as Christ's Last Supper was the 'entry to death.'[43] Since then the creative Son of God is in heaven *and* on earth: 'For where there is the body and blood of Christ, there Christ is. That is how it has been decided, that we should have it on earth. ... Just like the human being is of the earth and the earth is of him, so we are of Christ and Christ remains in us.'[44]

In his work on earth, and thus in the communion itself, Christ, the divine Logos, fulfilled the works of nature. According to Paracelsus he acted in the spirit of the spiritual cosmic order, but never in contradiction to nature whose real creator he is. Thus Christ was able to bring about physical healing through the power of his Word which is otherwise the preserve of natural processes. 'For he is the creator of medicine and thus the highest physician, and thus he has the greatest knowledge of nature.'[45]

Paracelsus composed his numerous writings on the communion in the few years around and following 1530, at a time when he had temporarily abandoned medicine to work exclusively as a theological lay preacher. Then he, who had walked in the sun of Christ, appears to have returned to practical medicine and medical writing, but now frequently arguing wholly on the basis of the gospels and Christology. Thus he wrote in a personal statement of justification in 1538:

> So I wish to defend myself for having produced and revealed a new medicine in accordance with the present rule. And if I were to be asked: Who taught you to do that? Do I ask you? Who teaches the leaves and grass to grow? For the same has said: come to me and learn from me for I am gentle and modest of heart. From it flows the foundation of truth.[46]

Through his work, Christ has renewed the eternal *and* the natural light — he has penetrated the earth and the heavens with his action and is thus as much 'teacher of the eternal' as he makes the plants grow and the physician develop.

Paracelsus' return to medicine will have been motivated, not least, by his unconditional will to heal; his powerful will to heal which he had always carried in his soul but which in turn may have experienced a far-reaching spiritual deepening through Christ in the key years about 1530. In 1538 he wrote:

> How can a physician say that a disease which is not deadly cannot be healed? ... Why do you not observe the sayings of Christ, who said: the sick require a physician? Are they not sick whom you reject? I say: yes. If they are sick, as it turns out, they require a physician. If they require a physician why do you say they cannot be helped?'[47]

The saying of Christ that the sick require a physician

from now on appears to have accompanied him wherever he went.

But his paths remained those of the loner who, largely misunderstood, continued to report about himself and his experiences but was little heard and even less taken seriously. Yet: 'How can I not appear strange to him who has never walked in the sun?'

Great Gospel, (c. 1000)

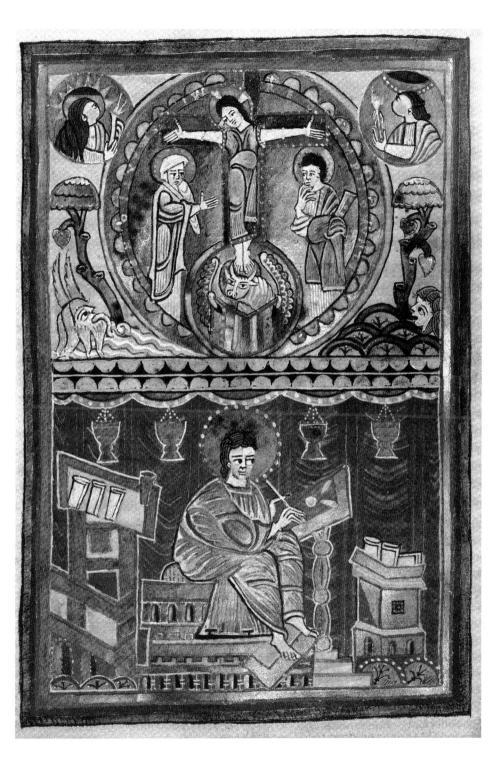

Rudolf Steiner

Experience fire *You walk with the Sun's beings*	Heat ♄
Experience air *You walk with the Sun's light*	Light ☉
Experience water *You walk with the Sun's action*	Chem. ☾
Experience the earth *You walk with the Sun's life* Rudolf Steiner[48]	♂ ☿

Rudolf Steiner, as scientist of the spirit, too walked 'in the Sun.' In his own words: 'My soul development depended on having stood in spirit before the mystery of Golgotha in innermost, utterly serious cognitive celebration.'[49] Steiner greatly respected the life achievement of the physician and spiritual natural scientist Paracelsus and in many instances paid tribute to his importance in world history.[50] He told anthroposophical physicians five years before his death:

> I myself ... would never present it as my profession, let us say, to discover something through the study of Paracelsus, but I sometimes have the strong desire to look up in Paracelsus how something is presented which I have discovered myself.[51]

Steiner worked at the establishment of a cosmological anthropology in the spirit of Christianity, something already intended by Paracelsus, in the context of the new Son mysteries right to his very last working period. Sustained witness to this is born, not least, by the so-called 'courses for young physicians.'[52]* Here Rudolf Steiner too accords key importance to the formation of physical substance and thus the continuing process of becoming human which extends as far as the dimension of the sacrament of communion and which was described by Rudolf Steiner in detail.

'Nature is permitted to become nature outside the human skin; within the human skin that which his nature turns into something that opposes nature.'[53] According to Rudolf Steiner, the human being possesses an 'organic tendency' to carry out directly 'the opposite somewhere of what is happening externally,'[54] thus establishing a 'wholly different world' — a world of 'organic internal processes' with its own laws. In this sense the healthy person radically transforms all the environmental qualities internalized by him, be it light and heat, be it nutritional substance. Here the necessary transformation process at the border between inner and outer world, or the active resistance of the autonomous inner world which brings it about forms the actual essential 'life process.'[55]* That is why Steiner also says with regard to nutrition: 'The reaction inside us against food is actually what we experience as the thing which stimulates us and sustains our life.'[56] And furthermore:

> Only when we understand how the organism is
> organized to receive stimuli to make it resistant ...
> only when we understand that the stimulus
> which produces the life process of nutrition lies in
> the resistance against [a substance] introduced

from the outside, will we be able to understand
nutrition properly. Nutrition is a process of resistance in that the ingestion of substances [should be
seen] only as an accompanying phenomenon by
means of which the stimulus to resistance is
guided into the finest reaches of the human being
from outside so that such resistance can extend
into the outer peripheral areas.[57]

If Paracelsus was already emphasizing that the internalization of food is connected with a breaking down
process, characterized as 'mouldiness,' which precedes
the 'new birth' of the substances in the human body, then
Rudolf Steiner too described the complete destruction or,
indeed, material elimination of the alien substance — he
spoke of its 'disappearance' — (taken into the gastro-
intestinal area) as the prerequisite for the 'resurrection of
new matter' which now belongs to the organism itself.[58]
Both processes — destruction and reconstruction, that is,
the extinguishing of all alien qualities *and* the revitalization of the substance, giving it soul and penetrating it with
spirit — are illustrated by Rudolf Steiner in his lectures on
spiritual science in a very concrete way, which we need
not go into further in this context.[59] Eventually they lead
to the formation of the blood as the central ego organ of
the human being and signify nothing less than nature
really 'becoming ego.'[60]

Here we must take into account that the overall process
of destruction, revitalization, ensouling and penetration
with ego-like spirit of internalized substance (or its
etheric, astral and ego penetration) involves the radical
suspension of earth forces in favour of the influence of *cosmic* forces. For the higher elements of the human being do
not work in the direction of earth but should rather be

seen as the individualized human organizational form of real cosmic forces. In the nutritional process they receive sustained and essential stimulus to be able to develop and strengthen their action in the body — a fact of spiritual science which Paracelsus may also have had in mind when he said that the 'inner firmament' was autonomous in terms of its forces and only required nutrition like a field requires manure. But here the real action of the human being's spiritual and cosmic elements in the substance require the complete destruction of the physical laws which previously applied in the substance — in the sense already characterized. Going beyond the nutritional process, Rudolf Steiner describes this repeatedly and in great detail, using the example of cosmically determined embryonic development, and in brief words also in respect of the homeopathic process which he, like Paracelsus, understood primarily as the suspension of physical laws with the subsequent action of higher entities.[61]*

Nutrition with earthly substances, Rudolf Steiner says, represent a process as a whole which causes the organism actively to defend itself — thus, however, bringing the higher, cosmically configured elements of the human being into play. Nevertheless, the new formation of physical substance as a consequence of the digestion process does not affect the organism as a whole, but merely concerns the nervous and sensory system. The material supply of the metabolic and limb system was described by Steiner as the expression of an original cosmic nutritional event. According to Steiner, the required active etheric qualities are internalized by human beings through a 'sensory and inhalation process':

A process is constantly taking place in the human being in which what is taken into the stomach flows upwards and is used in the head, and that what is taken into the head and the nervous and sensory system from the air and other environment flows downwards to become the organs of the digestive system or the limbs. If, therefore, you wish to know what the substance of your big toe consists of, you must not look at the nutrition. When you ask your brain, where does the substance come from, you must look at nutrition. But if you want to learn about the substance of your big toe, to the extent that it is not sensory substance imbued with heat and so on (to that extent it is nourished by the stomach), but if you wish to learn about the framework substance and so on, this is taken in through the breathing, the sensory organs, some of it even through the eyes. And all of these things ... pass into the organs in a seven-year cycle so that in terms of the substance of his limb and metabolic system, meaning the organs, the human being consists of cosmic substance. Only the nervous and sensory system is built up of telluric, of physical substance.'[62]

As a result of this physical and cosmic genesis, the continuing process of human development is an event of opposing flows of substance — upwards, through the physical stream of nutrition, the material of the nervous and sensory system is formed; downwards, from the cosmic environment, the matter of the metabolic and limb system. At the same time: 'What exists in the rhythmical part of the human being has an equalizing consequence in both directions.'[63]

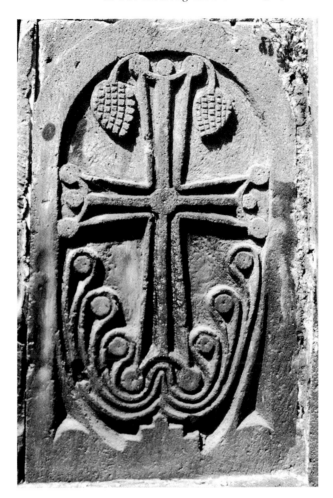

Stone cross at Kecharis Monastery (tenth century)

These mysterious connections in the way the human being is organized become even more profound when we further take into account that according to Rudolf Steiner's explanations there is a polar opposite relationship in the head and limb organization with regard to the *formative and functional forces*. Here the head is completely a cosmic organ of the heavens and the limbs are earthly tools, that is organs created by earth for the earth. So we can say overall:

> The head consists of earth substance and is formed in its plastic shape from the action of the heavens. The limbs of the human being, including the digestive system, are wholly shaped from the substance of the heavens. We would not see them if they were not flooded with physical substance by the head. But in walking, in grasping, in digesting, the substance of the heavens uses physical forces in order to live this life on earth from birth to death.[64]

In contrast, Steiner says about the mediating centre of the human being, about the rhythmical sphere of heart and lung:

> In the middle system, which comprises breathing and blood circulation, we have a mix of spiritual activity and material substance. The spiritual activity which flows through our breathing movement, our heart movement, is in turn accompanied by substance. And equally the substance of the physical being, to the extent that it flows into the breathing through oxygen, is accompanied by earthly activity. You can see, therefore, that everything flows together in the second system of the human being. Here heavenly substance and activity flow in, here physical activity and substance flow in.[65*]

The way that the human body is constructed from earth and cosmos, as well as their interaction in development and functions, are not ahistorical, eternal truths, according to Steiner, but are in turn embedded in a process of earth

and human development. Thus the central cosmic formation of substance in the metabolic and limb system really
only started on a sustained basis with the Christ event
which Rudolf Steiner described as the mystery of
Golgotha.[66] The healing middle sphere of the human
being also acquired its particular quality as a result. Here,
however, our observations flow into the spiritual sphere
of communion:

> Transubstantiation is placing into the external
> world what really happens in the innermost
> sphere of the human being. We see in transubstan-
> tiation what we cannot see in the external world
> because the external world is a fragment of exis-
> tence, not a totality. In the sacrament, we add that
> element to the external world which in the realm
> of nature is only fulfilled within the human
> being.[67]

Within the human being, in continuous human or ego
development, physical matter is fulfilled in the sense of
gradually turning to spirit. This is represented by the
sacrament. But in its real fulfilment — which according to
Rudolf Steiner was still seen as the 'highest alchemical
activity' in the twelfth and thirteenth centuries[68] — the
ego development of substance extends beyond the human
ego into the Christ ego; the process is subject directly to
the presence and action of Christ. Earth substance, originally from the sphere of the Father God, is taken into the
realm of the Son.

The unification of the human being with the spiritualized, dematerialized substance (communion) which in the
mass follows transubstantiation was described by Steiner
as a counter-process to the acquisition of physical characteristics by the human spirit soul whose incarnation

process requires adaptation to physical laws or partial adaptation to physical circumstances, requiring a constant counterbalance:

> The soul and spiritual element in human beings is faced at all times with the physical and bodily element; human beings must ensure that they get into the right rhythm to prevent the soul and spiritual element from becoming animalistic or that they do not ignore their physical side and descend into the soul and spiritual sphere in an unworldly way which weakens the soul and spirit. This is what human beings must seek to bring into a proper rhythm through receiving the sacrament at the altar.[69]

The broader horizon in terms of spiritual history of this sacramental and therapeutic balance was set out by Rudolf Steiner, following on from St Paul, who described Christ as the 'highest saviour of the soul in accordance with the rite of Melchizedek' (Heb.7:17, translation by Rudolf Steiner[70]). According to Steiner, Christ renewed at a higher level the historically preceding sacrificial offering of bread and wine of the priest king Melchizedek which at the time had already brought a key healing intervention into the situation of the incarnating human being. Melchizedek, Steiner explains, knew about the archetypal form of the sacrificial offering of bread and wine which contains a polar salt and sulphur (or sal and sulphur/phosphorous) principle and which can act in the spirit of an 'alchemy of salt and phosphorous' in the human being:

> What takes place ... in the human body — not outside the human body — through the combination of salt with phosphorous is a process which prop-

erly places the human being into earth existence
because the salt links him in the right way with
the earth whereas the phosphorous removes and
liberates him from earth existence in the proper
way. The human being who has salt and phosphorous within him the right way stands on earth in
the proper way, is strongly enough united with
earth but also contains the necessary etheric and
astral lightness to be free in his being of the earth
forces.[71]

The salt and sulphur effect practiced by Melchizedek —
which in detail can also be described as the healing force
to counter Luciferic divergence in the nervous and sensory system and Ahrmianic influences in the metabolic
and limb system — made it possible in terms of world history that human beings were capable of undergoing destiny at all.[72] Because this assumes that the moral quality of
a life on earth can be transferred to the subsequent incarnation and dealt with there:

Human beings cannot by themselves transfer into
their body without further ado what they have
undertaken in a life on earth, that is, they cannot
transfer it into the physical and etheric organization of the next life on earth; they can transfer it
— speaking now about the period before the mystery of Golgotha — if what takes place in the ritual with salt and phosphorous is undertaken on
their behalf as Melchizedek undertook the sacrificial offering of bread and wine. In this way
human beings in the period before the mystery of
Golgotha became capable of taking into the bodies
they received in their next life on earth the consequences of what they had done in the previous

life as good and bad deeds. In other words, this
was required if human beings were to develop
karma.[73]*

According to Steiner, the sacrificial rite of Melchizedek
was medicine for the sins of humankind in so far as it
enabled human beings to carry their sins with them to
resolve them in the future, that is to heal them. Thus the
essential errors did not fall prey to the 'Lord of this World'
who was described by Steiner as a 'spirit turned Luciferic
and Ahrimanic, particularly Ahrimanic'[74] and who would
have incorporated the concrete power of human evil into
the cosmic order if it had not been for the sacrificial deed
of the priest king Melchizedek.

According to Rudolf Steiner, Christ through the mystery
of Golgotha, the 'great sacrificial mass,' not only became
the 'master of karma' in continuation of Melchizedek as
well as in a great macrocosmic sense, accompanying and
ordering human destiny after death, making good and
healing the objective evil which occurred, without touching individual karmic responsibility.[75]* He also influenced
and continues to influence sacramentally the incarnated
human being through healing as the 'highest saviour of
the soul in accordance with the rite of Melchizedek.'
Steiner described in detail that it was and is the action of
Christ which countered the tendency of human beings to
incarnate too deeply, thus creating a balance to 'original
sin' — described by Steiner literally as an 'sickness.'[76]* The
Son god tears the human soul away from its ties to the
hereditary blood forces which at the time of Christ for the
first time threatened to occupy human consciousness as
such. 'In overcoming death on Golgotha, the forces were
created which can rekindle the lost forces in the human

soul.'[77] Physiologically, however, this action by Christ represents real intervention in the human physical structure. If up to the time of Christ the vital blood processes dominated, which according to Steiner derive their powers from the cosmically alive but physically dead nervous processes, the deed of Christ created a new harmonizing, freedom-building connection between both spheres:

> In having entrusted our nervous system to the earth for development, we entrusted it to death and left life above. This life we left above is the same which later followed in the being of Christ. The life of our nerves which we do not carry in us, which we have been unable to carry in us from the beginning of our existence on earth, followed in the Christ being. And what was there for this life to take hold of on earth? It had to take hold of the blood! Hence the focus on the mystery of the blood. What is divided in us in that the nervous system lost its cosmic life and the blood gained cosmic life, in that life became death and death became life, this achieved a new connection through the element which does not live in our physical nervous system descending from the cosmos, becoming human being, entering the blood and the blood uniting with the earth ... And we as human beings can balance out the contrast between our nervous system and blood system through participation in the mystery of Christ.[78]

In this sense the events of the sacrament affect and work in the essential core of the human being and from that basis establish the healing effect on the human being.[79]*

The centre of the human being is formed by the *heart* which rhythmically balances the divergent upper and lower poles of the body in collaboration with the breathing. When Ita Wegman questioned Rudolf Steiner, already in his sick bed, about the deeper spiritual background of the blood in the heart and lungs, Rudolf Steiner responded in writing. At the end of his explanation he wrote:

> What flows from the lungs to the heart is the
> human correlate of the descent of Christ to earth;
> the power flowing from the heart to the lungs is
> the human correlate of the passage of the human
> being after death into the spiritual world through
> the Christ impulse. To this extent the mystery of
> Golgotha lives in a human organic way between
> the heart and the lungs.[80]

In this sense the sacrament of communion as the continuing effect of the Christ event on Golgotha must also be considered as a central happening which is related to medicine. It is *healing medicine* because it heals and ensouls the human being in the core of his constitution; that is, it places him in the proper, spiritually appropriate relationship to the earth, thus strengthening him on the eternal path towards the good. If the sacramental event associated with the Logos extends as far as the human being and if it is able to develop its centring activity, it protects the soul against taking wrong paths which are often, or often become, paths of the body:

> When you have an insight into the mysterious
> connections between the insensitivity towards the
> Word, proclaiming the divine and the spiritual,
> and the problems with circulation and heart

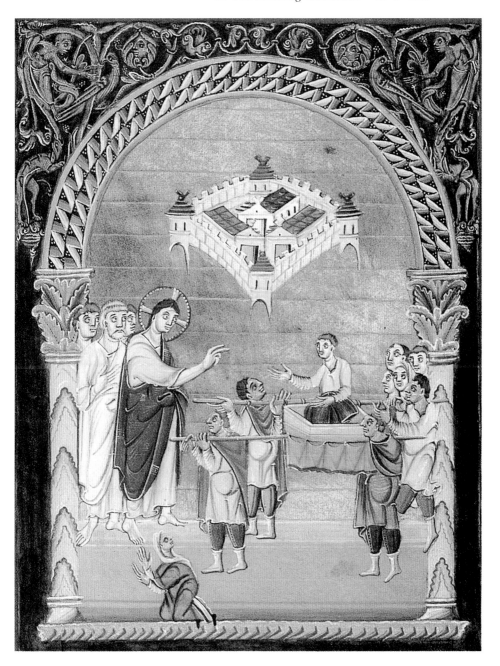

The healing of the young man of Nain (c. 1000)

> disease, and when you look at everything that
> rebounds — the pendulum not only swings away,
> it also swings back — in terms of materialistic
> views from the ruined blood circulation, the
> ruined heart as the result of such insensitivity
> towards the spirit-filled Word, then you will be
> able to judge the current situation of humanity;
> and then you will experience with the proper seri-
> ousness what religious renewal should actually
> be. Then you will also experience something of
> how the healing element can be found in the holy
> element and how healing does not need to be lost
> in the abstraction of sanctification.[81]

The medical and sacramental action of communion thus takes place in the border sphere between body and soul and concerns the whole basis of human incarnation; and it is in the latter that the basic diseases of the human being originate. According to Paracelsus and Rudolf Steiner, the historical Last Supper signified the 'first great stimulus for the approach of the realm of God through Christ'[82] and initiated a therapeutic and sacramental path intended to lead to the healing of the human being. In January 1924 Rudolf Steiner wrote down the following verse in his notebook:

You are soul
God's being is
Body in you

Your soul is
inhabited by spirit
Your body is
inhabited by spirit

Let God preside
in the body's spirit
And let egohood preside
in the soul's spirit

For if your soul's spirit
Takes your body's strength
You are sick in body
And if your body's spirit
Takes your soul's strength
You are sick in soul.[83]

4. The Soul Quickens in the Shrine of the Heart

The Human Heart as an Organ of Destiny

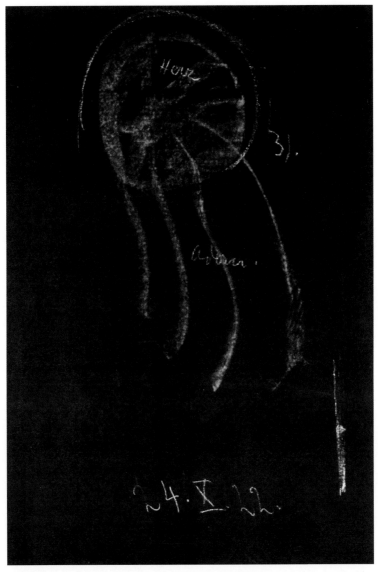

Blackboard drawing by Rudolf Steiner (Dornach, 1922)

Hearts interpret karma
When hearts learn to
Read the Word which
Forms
Human lives
When hearts learn to
Speak the Word which
forms
human essence.

Rudolf Steiner[1]

On his *own* sixty-third birthday, on February 27, 1924, Rudolf Steiner made a present of this verse to Ita Wegman together with a photograph. 'To my Mysa' he wrote under the lines.[2]

A verse which focuses on the *heart* as organ (*organon*, meaning instrument, tool) of karmic knowledge. The heart, Steiner said, is capable of *interpreting* karma in so far as it succeeds in perceiving the *Word* which is creatively active in *human life*, the Logos, and in reading its karmic script. But the experience of karma only becomes complete when the perceiving heart begins to speak the language of destiny itself, to speak the *Word* which is creatively active in the *human essence*. The receptive internalization of the laws of the senses on which human relationships depend is the (passive) first aspect of an understanding of destiny, the active side of which consists of the creative realization of the *Logos* — and is fulfilled in it.

On that day Rudolf Steiner gave this personal verse not just to someone who was linked to him in profound, ancient destiny; he also gave it to a woman who was a physician through and through and who for the whole of her life was in spiritual search of the *Word* which is *creatively active in the human essence* (in illness and in health). The verse gifted to Ita Wegman can therefore also be read and understood as witness of a developed spiritual ('esoteric') physiology; a physio-logy, a science of the Logos of the human physical body at whose centre is the *heart* and which Rudolf Steiner made accessible, showed and explained to Ita Wegman and other physicians in various contexts. 'Hearts interpret karma': we will see below the way in which Rudolf Steiner revealed the karmic dimension of the human heart, 'the soul quickening in the shrine of the heart.'

As early as 1911, Rudolf Steiner described the heart as the 'most noble' organ of the human being, as 'a kind of centre of the whole human organization.'[3] The heart mediates between the poles of the organism, it harmonizes the interaction between an 'upper' sphere of human existence oriented towards the environment (sensory perception, breathing) and those deep layers of the body in which the internalization and thus the individualizing transformation of external substance takes place (metabolism and blood formation). External world and internal world, 'you' (environment and other people) and 'I' (sense of self) meet in the heart, find and develop here their unique centre.

Years later Steiner expanded this for the physicians with the remark that such harmonizing mediation by the heart takes place essentially via an act of *perception*. The

heart, Steiner said, is a 'sensory organ which is internalized to a high degree'; through this organ the nervous
and sensory processes of the upper human being can perceive, indeed, experience what happens in the depths of
the body, in the organic processes of the lower human
being.[4] Steiner wrote in his notebook: 'It transforms what
happens in the metabolic organs, turns this into content
which can be experienced.'[5] The 'upper' transforms the
'lower,' ensouls it, 'turns it into content which can be
experienced.' But that also means that the head structure,
formed out of the temporal dynamic of the past, witness
of biographical memory, perceives the life lived in the
present through the organ of the heart, internalizes the
current happenings in life and turns them into ego-filled,
future-oriented life stories. The action of the blood — as
Rudolf Steiner explained in his lectures about Thomas
Aquinas at Whitsun 1920 — is exemplified in the motion
of the heart; the activity of the heart is taken into 'the
whole of the human individual.'[6]

Although not particularly emphasized by Rudolf Steiner
in this way, the physiological descriptions of the heart
(from 1911 to 1920) which have been sketched out so far
did already contain something of the deeper spiritual
background which gradually illustrated the heart as the
central organ of the human life story. The heart is not a
'pump' and does not govern the circulation; on the contrary, the activity of the blood as the expression of the
current life process is perceived ('read') by it and
'answered,' that is brought into harmony with the
requirements of the past and the future and thus harmo-
nized in terms of time.

In two lectures of July 1921 and May 1922 Rudolf

Steiner then dealt quite explicitly with the heart as the organ of destiny — as the organ of a life story which transcends biography. On May 26, 1922 he outlined for the first time the transformation of the heart in terms of developmental physiology at the time of puberty, of *physical maturity*. During this transitional period from childhood to youth there arises in the cosmically configured life body a centralized organ of the heart with etheric substance. It replaces a preceding organ which was formed out of the forces of the physical organization. This newly formed etheric heart is able to take in those (astral) forces which develop in the soul body due to the actions we take and are inscribed in it. In this way the cosmic etheric forces combine at the time of puberty with those earthly developments arising from the deeds and suffering of the human being: 'In the region of the heart there is a fusion of the cosmic with the earthly, and it takes place in such a way that the cosmic is taken into the etheric in its cosmic configuration and prepares there to take in all our deeds, everything we do.'[7]

As the ego increasingly combines with the heart-centred blood circulation at the approach of puberty, the spiritual background and individual intentions of our acts of will are included in the developing cardiac 'organism of karmic development.'[8] Thus as we enter into youth, the 'most noble' organ of the human being arises anew and individually; from puberty onwards it enables the future-oriented internalization of life as it is lived and thus the real development of destiny which is subject to our own responsibility. The completed life process is taken into the core of the human being, 'into the whole human individuality.'

In the heart the actions (and motives for action) of the human being are 'spiritualized,' Steiner said on July 2, 1921 in Dornach.[9] Inside the organ of the heart, in its 'incredibly fine heat structures,' the transformed forces of the metabolic and limb system collect which are connected with human actions (and their relationships).[10] The heart is 'the organ which carries from the metabolic and limb organism, through the mediation of the metabolic and limb organism, what we understand as karma into the next incarnation.'[11] As Steiner responded in writing to the question from Ita Wegman, 'How is future karma related to the heart?' the heart is involved 'in the formation of karma only to the extent that it is part of the metabolic and limb organism.'[12] In the heart, the 'karmic predispositions,' the concrete and specific impulses for the future, are prepared on the basis of spiritualized motives and actions:

> When you look into your heart, you can see pretty well — in outline, not as a fully filled in picture — what you will do in your next life. We can therefore say not just in general, *in abstracto,* that we prepare in our current life what will have a karmic effect in the next one, but we can directly show the casket, I might say, which contains the karma of future periods.[13]

In the New Testament, Matthew says:

> Do not collect earthly treasures, for they are eaten up by moths and rust, and thieves rummage through them and steal them. Rather, gather treasures in the spiritual world. They cannot be eaten by moths and rust, nor can thieves rummage through them and steal them. Where you have gathered a treasure, thither you heart forces will bear you. (Matt.6:19–21).[14*]

In the heart
Lives an element of the human being
Which of all of them
Contains substance
Which is the most spiritual;
Which of all of them
Lives spiritually
In the way which is
Most physically revealed.
Hence the Sun
In the human cosmos is
The heart;
Hence in the heart
The human being
Is utmost
In his being's
Deepest source.[15]

In 1924, Rudolf Steiner wrote: 'The age of Michael has commenced. Hearts begin to have thoughts.'[16] Such thinking of the heart, which also repeatedly comes to expression in the gospel document, may possibly be a further building block for understanding the poetic verse, which Rudolf Steiner gave to Ita Wegman on February 27, 1924. The 'interpretation of karma' by the heart, the 'reading' and, in particular, the 'speaking' of the Word can also be understood as a process in the Michaelic thinking which is undertaken in the communication between brain and heart. Michael, Steiner wrote in the same essay, 'liberates the thoughts from the sphere of the head; he clears their way to the heart.' In 1911, Rudolf Steiner not only held the first major course about spiritual ('esoteric') physiology in Prague, but also for the first time revealed (in it) insights into the physiological interaction of the heart and the brain — referring to the 'etherization of the blood.' In the heart, Steiner said, the substance of the blood etherizes and creates a current to the brain.

On October 1, 1911, Rudolf Steiner hinted in Basle that this rarefied blood flow in the human being is able to combine with the 'flow of blood of Christ' which impregnated the earth as the result of the event of the mystery of Golgotha and which has also undergone an etherization process: 'And just as our blood flows as ether from the heart upwards, so the etherized blood of Jesus Christ has lived in the earth's ether since the mystery of Golgotha.' The effect of the etherized blood of Christ can also act in the rising human blood flow, Steiner says, except:

> A connection between both streams can only be established if the human being understands the content of the Christ impulse in the right way. Otherwise a connection cannot be established, otherwise both streams repel one another.'[17]

If, however, the work of Christ is understood in the right way — that is with the perceptual possibilities given by the new, etheric revelation of Christ — the rising etherization of the blood combines with the substantive power of the Logos.

In his Whitsun lectures on the philosophy of Thomas Aquinas, the *Doctor eximius* whom Benozzo Gozzoli once painted with a shining golden heart, Steiner spoke about the necessary Christianization of the human thinking, about the *redemption* of the thinking.[18] If this depiction is taken together with the Basle outline of a spiritual physiology of October 1, 1911, then the sacrificial deed of Christ,

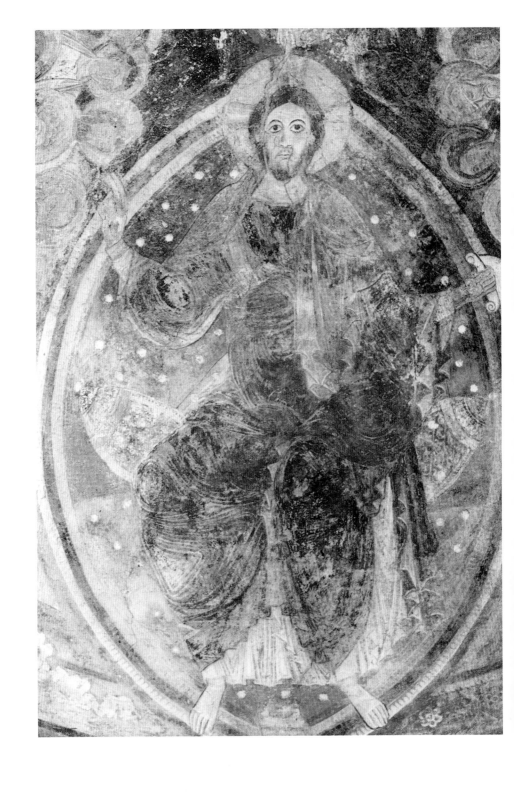

his substantial karmic connection with the earth, can be understood as the prerequisite for the kind of Michaelic *redeemed* thinking of the heart whose risen spirituality supports the evolution of the world and is associated with an increasing understanding of destiny. The *speaking* of the *Word* which completes the *interpretation of karma* is then a unique Christological fact and points to the action in terms of a spiritual physiology of him who *bears and orders* human destiny. The thinking of the heart becomes visible as the spiritual thinking of the future. It takes place in the light and with the assistance of the risen Logos, *sub species reincarnationis et aeternitatis.*

> Hearts interpret karma
> When hearts learn to
> Read the Word
> That is creative
> in human life
> When hearts learn to
> Speak the Word
> That is creative
> in human essence.

Majestas Domini (Berzé-la-Ville Abbey, c. 1100)

Endnotes

GA   Rudolf Steiner's Complete Works (Gesamtausgabe)

1. From Helene von Grunelius' estate (Ita Wegman Archive, Arlesheim)

Introduction

1. GA 266, p. 133f.
2. Wegman, *Das Mysterium der Erde.* On Rudolf Steiner's collaboration with Ita Wegman see Zeylmans van Emmichoven, *Wer war Ita Wegman.*

1. Et Incarnatus Est

1. GA 123, p. 188.
2. Compare Rudolf Frieling's interpretation on the healing of the blind and the healing of the deaf and dumb man in *Christologische Aufsätze,* pp. 217ff and 202ff.
3. For example Luke 10:17: 'The seventy returned and said joyfully, "Lord, even the demons obey us through the power of your name!"'
4. GA 123, p. 191.
5. GA 114, p. 206.
6. Kienle, *Christentum und Medizin,* p. 8.
7. See Kienle, *Die Krankenpflege im Abendland.*
8. GA 28, p. 272. Rudolf Steiner spoke about the central significance of such an experience of Christ for modern spiritual medicine in his London lecture of November 16, 1922 (GA 218). The lecture also gives an indication of the subtle spiritual prerequisites required for the Raphael School which, as medical mystery school of the twentieth century, was established as late as September 1924 following a long period of consideration by Rudolf Steiner. 'It is not that simple; it

must be wanted by the spiritual world and there must be people who want to receive it.' Quoted from Zeylmans van Emmichoven, *Wer war Ita Wegman*, p. 217.

9. GA 318, p. 163.
10. Deventer, *Die anthroposophisch-medizinische Bewegung*, p. 29f.
11. Notebook belonging to Ita Wegman, quoted in Zeylmans van Emmichoven, *Wer war Ita Wegman*, p. 217.
12. GA 114, p. 165.
13. This and following two quotations from GA 123, p. 187.
14. Gerhard Kienle established in 1981 *(Christentum und Medizin)* and 1983 *(Die ungeschriebene Philosophie Jesu)* that the healing processes in the New Testament can be philosophically understood on the basis of the Platonic and Aristotelian way of thinking and represent a further radicalization of the classical understanding of therapy.

In the Platonic view, the soul as formative principle preserves the order of the body but is always in tension between the divine spiritual world of ideas and the disintegrating sphere of matter. Developing ideas of Konrad Gaiser *(Platons ungeschriebene Lehre)*, Kienle writes: 'In the end it lies within the volition of the soul itself to decide whether to turn towards the world of ideas, to its forms and the world form or God, or whether to give itself over to *kakia* or disintegration which rules pure matter. By turning towards the highest form accessible to it, to the *nous* or the divine spirit, the soul gains the strength to "shift" its state and that of its body in such a way that the comprehensive form of the body can be re-established from the given opportunities. In such a moral and physical restoration the soul connects to the cosmic order which lies in God. The expression "repent" (Matt.3:2) thus becomes doubly comprehensible: the soul makes the free decision to turn away from *kakia* in matter to the *nous*' *(Die ungeschriebene Philosophie Jesu,* p. 39).

According to Kienle, the encounter between Christ and the sick people led to the reconnection of the soul with the divine world order, to a healing process in the sense of 'finding one's proper relationship with the world order'

(Christentum und Medizin, p. 47). Christ enables such a movement of soul of the sick person to the *nous,* the divine ground of the world of the Father, for: 'The exceptionally strong power to set things moving of Jesus' spirit-filled soul affected other souls and through their souls their bodies' *(Christentum und Medizin,* p. 41).

15. GA 139, p. 65.
16. GA 114, p. 186.
17. Rittelmeyer, *Briefe über das Johannesevangelium,* p. 342.
18. GA 114, p. 185.
19. GA 114, p. 166ff. See also the notable work of the priest Karl Hublow (1901–79) on the healing frescoes in St George's church on the Island of Reichenau with regard to the anthropological aspects of individual cases of healing in the gospels.
20. In contrast to the two other people 'raised from the dead' in the New Testament, Lazarus and the youth of Nain, which were described by Steiner as 'initiation processes' and not as the healing of sickness, he understood the raising of the daughter of Jairus as a proper healing process. According to Steiner, the daughter of the Jewish leader of the synagogue in Capernaum was only 'close to death' (GA 114 (The Gospel of St Luke), p. 170).
21. GA 100, p. 260.
22. GA 114, p. 171.
23. GA 139, p. 68f. In 1946, Emil Bock pointed out in his major book on the activities of Christ between the baptism in Jordan and the mystery of Golgotha *(The Three Years)* that the disciples summoned by Christ for the healing of the daughter of Jairus, Peter, James and John, were also present at the transfiguration on Mount Tabor where they gained insight into a further karmic relationship, the connection between the individuality of Elijah and the appearance of John the Baptist: 'Then the disciples *understood* that he was speaking to them of John the Baptist.' (Matt.17:13, author's emphasis). Bock wrote about this: 'In the teaching which Jesus gave to the three as he returned with them from the mount of transfiguration, he allowed ... the cognitive seeds

to grow which were placed into the souls of these disciples at Jairus' house. ... Undoubtedly the intimate instruction in karma which Jesus gave to the three disciples in the aftermath of the Tabor experiences was much more detailed than is revealed in the gospel, which only reproduces the sequence of events in outline. Perhaps at that hour the idea of repeated earth lives was also applied to the riddle which the disciples had been allowed to witness in Jairus' house.' (*Die drei Jahre*, p.243f.)

24. GA 114, p. 166.
25. GA 114, p. 188.
26. Frieling, *Christologische Aufsätze*, p.225ff.
27. 'Then the neighbours and those who had seen him before as a blind beggar, said, "Is that not the man who used to sit and beg?" Others said, "Yes, it is." And yet others said, "No, he only looks like him." *Then he himself spoke, "I am that man"* (John 9:8f). Rudolf Frieling pointed out that this is the only place in the New Testament in which the divine phrase, the divine 'I am' *(ego eimi)* of the gospels passes the lips of a *human being*. Peter, by contrast, loses his the power of his individuality in the course of this threefold denial of Christ — Luke and John have him speak the words *I am not*. In the version of Matthew Peter is quoted in this context as saying: *I do not know the man* (Matt.26:74). We might say that Peter loses his essential humanness on losing the dimension of Christ in his own being.
28. GA 143, p.184.
29. GA 133, p. 116.
30. Rittelmeyer, *Meine Lebensbegegnung mit Rudolf Steiner*, p. 76f.
31. Rittelmeyer, *Meine Lebensbegegnung mit Rudolf Steiner*, p.78.
32. Compare: 'Every morning we — there were about forty [34] participants — attended Steiner's lecture in the studio building in a celebratory and joyful mood.' (F. Husemann quoted in Selg, *Anfänge anthroposophischer Heilkunst*, p. 90). But according to O. Schmiedel, the first medical course mostly took place in the Glass House. (Schmiedel, 'Aufzeichnungen,' in Zeylmans van Emmichoven, *Wer war Ita Wegman*, Vol. 3, pp. 414–61.) Whether lectures were held

in both places, whether Husemann was possibly referring to the 'glass studio' or whether other circumstances prevailed cannot be determined with any certainty at present.

33. Zeylmans van Emmichoven, *Willem Zeylmans van Emmichoven*, p. 79.

34. GA 317, p. 203.

35. Compare Zeylmans van Emmichoven, *Wer war Ita Wegman*, Vol. 1, pp. 155ff and Vol. 2, pp. 374f.

36. Compare Zeylmans van Emmichoven, *Wer war Ita Wegman*, Vol. 2, p. 253, and Selg, *Der Engel über dem Lauenstein*.

37. Nik Fiechter, 'Eine Heilmeditation für ein Kind,' pp. 43f.

38. The archetypal image of this healing process can be found, once again, in the gospels. Many of Christ's healing acts only found completion in the Temple. There, in the inner space of the sacred building, Christ 'found' the sick person again and deepened the consciousness aspect of his healing through the spoken word: 'See, you have become well.' (John 5:14).

39. A.G. Degenaar, *Krankheitsfälle und andere medizinische Fragen*, p. 25 (Patient 41).

2. From Empathy with Suffering to Karmic Resolve

1. Deventer, 'Ita Wegmans Wirken als Arzt,' Quoted from Zeylmans van Emmichoven, *Wer war Ita Wegman*, Vol. 2, p. 337.

2. Rudolf Steiner, October 21, 1917, quoted from Fant, Klingborg, Wilkes, *Die Holzplastik Rudolf Steiners in Dornach*, p. 21. One year later (September 21, 1918), Rudolf Steiner said that the Goetheanum represented a 'state of equilibrium in the cosmos' removed from the realms of Lucifer and Ahriman, and: 'Everything climaxes in the central figure of our group, in the representative of humankind, in whom everything Luciferic and Ahrimanic is to be extinguished' (GA 184, p. 170).

3. 'Great intellectuality in the med course lectures ... my surprise about such intellectuality,' Ita Wegman notes looking back in a draft lecture paper (London, January 27, 1932), and in a notebook she records a few years later one of her

questions to Rudolf Steiner in summer 1923 in Penmaen-
mawr: 'Why do the medical courses have to be made so
intellectual?' (Quoted from Zeylmans van Emmichoven,
Wer war Ita Wegman, Vol. 1, p. 290 and Vol. 2, p. 216.) It
must be taken into account here, however, that Wegman's
surprise was related to the tone of the medical lectures from
1920 to 1923. In the first course for young physicians which
started on January 2, 1924, she then experienced the first
fulfilment of her longing over many years for a different
way of presentation by Rudolf Steiner which took account
of the therapeutic attitude of the physician and thus the
courage to heal, the *will to heal* and *karmic resolve* together
with the presentation of a cosmologically deepened esoteric
medicine.

4. GA 317, pp. 203ff.
5. GA 114, p. 185f.
6. GA 120, p. 202.
7. Compare Selg, 'Die Medizin im Lebensgang Rudolf
   Steiners,' as well as 'Eine kurze Skizze der Geschichte der
   anthroposophischen Medizin bis zum Tod Rudolf Steiners',
   in Selg, *Anthroposophische Ärzte,* p. 25ff. With regard to the
   exemplary debate with the physicians at the Clinic and
   Therapeutic Institute in Stuttgart, compare Selg, *Anfänge
   anthroposophischer Heilkunst,* p. 98ff.
8. GA 268, p. 195. Compare also Steiner, 'Das Geheimnis der
   Wunde,
9. 'Matthew says expressly that Jesus was gripped by a *deep
   compassion. On that basis* he touched their eyes and they
   received sight' (Frieling, *Christologische Aufsätze,* p. 218).
10. Ita Wegman Archive, (Arlesheim). According to Hilma
    Walter, Ita Wegman received this verse from Rudolf Steiner
    on December 2, 1923 for the nurses in the Clinic in
    Arlesheim. The meditation was most recently published in
    a wording diverging from Wegman's handwritten text and
    dated 1924/5 by the Rudolf Steiner Nachlassverwaltung
    (GA 268, p. 310). The version of the meditation printed
    there goes: *In the heart lives / The shining brightness / Of the
    human being's / sense of helping / In the heart is active / In*

warming strength / The human being's helping power */ So let us carry / The soul's full will /* In *the heart's warmth / And the heart's light / Thus we* bring */ Salvation /* Through *God's mercy / To those in need of healing.*

11. In GA 268, p.194.

12. GA 316, p. 141.

13. GA 316, p. 220

14. It should, however, be taken into account with regard to the possible correspondence between the *will to heal* and the *will to recover* that Rudolf Steiner squarely placed responsibility for the development of the former therapeutic dimension of will with the physician (and *not* the patient). It requires the physician's developed will to heal for the patient's will to recover to develop almost like a reflex. Current psychotherapy turns this relationship on its head — here it is the so-called 'unmotivated' patient who (on top of his illness) also carries responsibility for the possibly unsuccessful (because 'unwanted') treatment.

15. With regard to this will dimension of true cognitive *action* see also the writings of Gerhard Kienle which were posthumously edited by his friend, Rev. Diether Lauenstein, *Die ungeschriebene Philosophie Jesu.*

16. This *warmth* meditation, the preparation of which contains guidance towards the *will* part of the human soul, leads to the experience by the physician of Christ in the etheric, according to Rudolf Steiner. If it is practiced, the spirit which was to work in the new anthroposophical medicine, which was to stand spiritually behind the *will to heal,* becomes apparent.

    Helene von Grunelius (1897–1936) later became a great anthroposophical physician and clearly practiced her teacher's Christian will to heal in an exemplary manner (see the beginning of this book). She died in Ita Wegman's clinic in Arlesheim at the early age of thirty-nine. 'When I visited her a short time before her death at Burghalde, she said in the course of the long talks we had during our walks that she now felt able to cope with any illness.' (Deventer, *Die anthroposophisch-medizinische Bewegung,* p. 24.)

17. GA 317, p. 165.
18. GA 317, p. 166.
19. GA 317, p. 122.
20. GA 314, p. 283.
21. In a short note, Steiner reports on April 22, 1924 that at the age of 22 (that is, in about 1883 in Vienna) he had put himself in close proximity to a woman suffering from smallpox since he was tutoring her son in the sick room (only separated by a screen). Steiner added: 'But I did that with pleasure also in order to see how one can protect oneself' (GA 314, p. 287). It may be assumed that in precisely this situation Steiner studied smallpox from the perspective of spiritual science — in May 1910 he emphasized in Hamburg that the findings imparted there about individual clinical pictures (including smallpox) had been acquired from concrete cases. 'I must repeat in this context that only such examples [of diseases] have been given which have been investigated on the basis of spiritual science; these are not hypotheses but cases. That is why you cannot demand that they are exhaustive, because I am not setting up hypotheses but cases which must be taken as such' (GA 120, p. 120).
22. GA 317, p. 116.
23. Kienle, *Die Zeitlage im Verhältnis zu Raphael und Michael.*
24. GA 120, p. 83.
25. GA 312, p. 346.
26. GA 312, p. 190 and GA 313, p. 115.
27. GA 312, p. 379. In this context it should also be taken into account that *all* 34 participants at the first medical course were members of the Anthroposophical Society and Rudolf Steiner could clearly assume some knowledge among his listeners of the spiritual background to his presentation.
28. GA 74, p. 108.
29. GA 74, p. 104.
30. GA 314, p. 281.
31. GA 316, p. 204.
32. S.J. Pollock, 'Clinical trials.'
33. Kienle, *Die Zeitlage im Verhältnis zu Raphael und Michael.*
34. Such a medicine based in Christianity implies the ability of

the individual physician to perceive the sick person as an individual and to *recognize* the disease processes as events connected with changes in the different components that make up the human being. To this extent it assumes that the sick person is *understood,* accepted and supported in concrete terms as the physical incarnation of a soul and spirit. As Gerhard Kienle puts it: 'Thus we can say, medicine based in Christianity is a type of medicine which requires that the human being can find himself as a comprehensive individuality, which requires discovering and acknowledging the comprehensive individuality in the other and *reflecting* on its relationship with events in the physical body.' (*Christentum und Medizin,* p. 90, my emphasis). In his *Ungeschriebene Jahre Jesu,* Kienle develops the idea among other things that the promotion of the individual human capacities and abilities for cognition are also a central theme in the gospels: 'If you can live and find permanence in my word, then you really are my disciples, and you will recognize the truth, and the truth will lead you to freedom' (John 8:31f). According to Kienle, the radical insight of the individual disciple, extending as far as cognition of history, human nature and destiny, was the purpose of Jesus' teaching; his listeners were individually to become capable or making judgments and decision independently of the general opinion, the consensus of the majority.

35. GA 316, p. 205.
36. GA 316, p. 205.
37. GA 316, p. 121.
38. GA 316, pp. 86, 122.
39. GA 316, p. 86
40. GA 131, p. 78ff. See also GA 130, lectures of September 21 and December 2, 1911.
41. GA 120, p. 112.
42. GA 145, p. 164.
43. GA 150, p. 25.
44. GA 145, p. 161. A 'macrocosmic protective impulse' is how Steiner characterizes the physical incarnation of Christ at the turning point in time (with regard to Ahriman) and the

coming appearance of Christ in the etheric (with regard to Lucifer) — see GA 145, p.163.

45. GA 120, p. 217.

46. The meditation *The human being is a bridge / Between the past and the existence of the future ...,* which Rudolf Steiner wrote down on December 24, 1920 and which was found in Ita Wegman's estate (GA 40, p. 143), is a key Christian one in the context of the background set out here. Lucifer and Ahriman want to destroy this bridge through a one-sided fixation on the spiritual past (Lucifer) or alternatively on the non-historical, materialized present (Ahriman) which, of course, has no future either (compare GA 203, lecture of March 11, 1921).

47. GA 158, p. 120.

48. GA 158, lecture of November 21, 1914, and GA 156, lecture of December 13, 1914.

49. GA 170, lectures of September 2 and 3, 1916. References to the action of Lucifer and Ahriman in the course of the individual developmental physiology of the first seven years in a person's life were particularly made by Steiner in his Augsburg lecture of March 14, 1913 (GA 150).

50. GA 169, p. 42.

51. For details on a physiological level see Selg, *Vom Logos menschlicher Physis,* pp. 505ff.

52. GA 210, p. 14.

53. GA 211, p. 192.

54. GA 203, p. 260, and GA 177, p. 65.

55. See GA 191, lecture of November 1, 1919. Here Rudolf Steiner describes in detail how such preparation is currently being undertaken.

56. GA 211, p.206.

57. GA 316, p. 205.

58. GA 120, p.139f.

59. See for instance Rudolf Steiner's statement of 1910: 'It would, in the spirit of what I myself would consider to be the spiritual scientific movement, be my most urgent wish that those who have a physiological and medical training familiarize themselves with the facts to such an extent that

they could examine physiology with regard to its factual character.' (GA 125, p. 89.) That this most urgent wish of Rudolf Steiner's was not even begun to be fulfilled emerges clearly from the following sentences spoken in October 1917: 'Oh, I made a lot of effort to encourage such people to make the connection. What indeed might have been if a physiology, a biology with all the specialist knowledge which can be acquired in these fields today had spiritually worked through physiology and biology so that, without necessarily using our terms, work had been undertaken in these individual sciences in our spirit!' (GA 177, p.176).

60. See Selg, *Gerhard Kienle*, pp. 295–356.

61. Kienle, *Die Zeitlage*. On the 'demons of Bacon' compare Rudolf Steiner's lecture of September 16, 1924 (GA 328).

62. GA 74, p. 95.

63. Quoted from Gisbert Husemann, 'Lili Kolisko.'

64. GA 260, p. 210.

65. GA 120, p. 112.

66. Hamburg, GA 118. St Gallen, GA 178, p. 72. London GA 218.

67. GA 211, p. 209f.

68. GA 120, p. 169.

69. As Steiner explained to the physicians, this also implies that the physician himself is willing to refrain from the action of medicines in his own organic diseases (compare GA 316, p. 101f.).

70. Gerhard Kienle, *Die Zeitlage*.

71. Steiner here directly characterizes *types* of Ahrimanic and Luciferic illnesses and also describes typologically appropriate treatment methods adapted to the dimensions of Lucifer and Ahriman (such as applied heat or coldness versus the therapeutic use of electricity) and adds: 'If that were taken into account, the right principles would also be found for giving the appropriate help to the sick person.' (GA 120, p. 88)

72. This spiritual side of the process of overcoming the illness had been repeatedly discussed by Steiner as early as 1909 in close connection with first accounts of Lucifer and Ahriman

(compare *Geisteswissenschaftliche Menschenkunde,* GA 107, lecture of January 26, 1909, and *Der Christus-Impuls und die Entwicklung des Ich-Bewußtsein,* GA 116, lecture of December 22, 1909).

73. From Helene von Grunelius' estate (see dedication, p. 9)
74. This applies not just to Steiner's spiritual scientific research in the field of illness but also with regard to the understanding of medicines. An indication in this respect can be found in the lecture of October 25, 1915, where he says: 'But only those will be able to fertilize medicine in the right way with the guidelines of spiritual science who are not afraid to penetrate the veil of nature so that they enter the Ahrimanic world and have to fight against the spirits of destruction. In order to find what heals human beings, we have to enter the region of those spirits who dissolve everything in the human being which causes illness and death, for only where the deeper causes of death and illness can be found can the medicines be sought.' (GA 254, p. 192.)
75. GA 218, p. 154.
76. GA 218, pp. 157–59.
77. See Frieling, *Christologische Aufsätze,* p. 225ff. In relation to this healing account see also Rudolf Steiner's lecture of July 2, 1909 (GA 112).

3. The Healing Medicine

1. Benjamin, *Das Passagenwerk,* p. 637.
2. In this respect see, for instance, the statements by Rudolf Steiner: 'The key thing is that the whole meaning of Christianity lives in the ritual of the sacrifice of the mass.' And: 'The Christian stream is always immediately present in the Act of Consecration of Man ... and this stream of Christian substance moves through the Act of Consecration of Man so that actually this Act of Consecration of Man should be at the centre of Christian ritual' (GA 343, p. 474, and GA 344, p. 452).
3. GA 344, p.223.
4. GA 216, p. 20.
5. Wolfram von Eschenbach, *Parzival,* Vol. 2, Book 19.

6. Quoted from Sudhoff, *Theophrast von Hohenheim,* Section I, Vol. 9, p. 71.
7. Of Paracelsus' writings on the communion only the text *The Lord's Supper (De coena domini libri VII ad Clementem VV. Papam)* has appeared in print. The anthroposophist Gerhard Deggeller (1908–95), German scholar and collaborator on the Heidelberg Paracelsus Edition, published this work with a commentary independently in 1950 together with Paracelsus' interpretation of the Lord's Prayer. Deggeller's edition of the communion writings is based on a copy from the original Wolfenbüttel manuscript (Herzog August Library).
8. Pörksen, 'Konturen des Ich.'
9. Peuckert, *Theophrastus Paracelsus. Werke,* Vol. I, p. 200.
10. Peuckert, Vol. 2, p. 38.
11. Peuckert, Vol. 1, p. 561.
12. Peuckert, Vol. 1, p. 544.
13. Peuckert, Vol. 1, p. 545.
14. Peuckert, Vol. 1, p. 548f.
15. Peuckert, Vol. 1, p. 552.
16. Peuckert, Vol. 1, p. 554.
17. Peuckert, Vol. 1, p. 208f.
18. Peuckert, Vol. 1, p. 214.
19. Peuckert, Vol. 1, p. 210.
20. Peuckert, Vol. 1, p. 76.
21. Peuckert, Vol. 2, p. 33f (my emphasis).
22. Peuckert, Vol. 2, p. 34.
23. Peuckert, Vol. 2, p. 32.
24. Peuckert, Vol. 2, p. 36.
25. Peuckert, Vol. 2, pp. 33, 36.
26. Peuckert, Vol. 2, p. 34.
27. Deggeller, *Paracelsus,* pp. 61f.
28. Peuckert, Vol. 2, p. 35.
29. Sudhoff, Vol. 12, p. 32.
30. Sudhoff, Vol. 8, p. 100.
31. Peuckert, Vol. 2, p. 37.
32. Peuckert, Vol. 2, p. 38,
33. Degeller, *Paracelsus,* p. 45

34. Degeller, *Paracelsus*, p. 62f.
35. Degeller, *Paracelsus*, p. 62.
36. Degeller, *Paracelsus*, p. 54.
37. Degeller, *Paracelsus*, p. 51.
38. Degeller, *Paracelsus*, p. 55.
39. Degeller, *Paracelsus*, p. 15.
40. Degeller, *Paracelsus*, p. 56.
41. Degeller, *Paracelsus*, p. 37.
42. Degeller, *Paracelsus*, p. 40.
43. Degeller, *Paracelsus*, p. 30.
44. Degeller, *Paracelsus*, pp. 41f./33.
45. Degeller, *Paracelsus*, p. 58.
46. Peuckert, Vol. 2, p. 500.
47. Peuckert, Vol. 2, p.501.
48. GA 268, p. 300.
49. GA 28, p. 272.
50. See Selg, 'Die Paracelsus-Rezeption Rudolf Steiners.'
51. GA 312, p. 208.
52. In the overall context consider Steiner's statement: 'It is certainly true to say that there were mighty teachings about Christianity in the writings denounced as Gnostic and in other older accounts of the ancient teachers of the Church who had still been pupils of the Apostles or pupils of the Apostles' pupils. Such teachings were then eradicated by the Church because the Church wanted to get rid of what was always associated with such teachings: the cosmic aspect. Immensely important things have been destroyed by the Church. They have been destroyed, but study of the Akashic record will restore them down to the last dot on the i when the time has come to restore them.' (GA 346, p. 129).
    In his courses for young physicians, Rudolf Steiner revealed to the students and physicians the 'original cosmic way of thinking about the human being' (GA 316, p. 194) which existed in ancient medical practice and was intimately connected with esoteric Christianity. With it is associated a pronounced 'dedicated behaviour of the soul in the world' (GA 316, p. 197) which also means that the 'Christian

will to heal' (compare p. 47ff) expressly implemented by
Rudolf Steiner cannot be separated at all from the 'original
cosmic way of thinking about the human being'. Against
this background we can also consider the following meditation, which Rudolf Steiner gave his young listeners: 'Feel in
the fever's measure / The spiritual gift of Saturn / Feel in
the pulse's number / The Sun's strength of soul / Feel in the
weight of matter / The Moon's formative power / Then you
will see in your will to heal / Also what needs to be healed
in the human beings on earth' (GA 316, pp. 200f).

Incidentally, Paracelsus, too, expressly put his faith in
young physicians with regard to the Christian will to heal
and thus with regard to his whole medical reforms.
Around 1530 he wrote in explanation: 'It is a characteristic
of the light of nature that it enters the human being in the
cradle, that it is beaten into him with a rod, that it is
dragged close up by the hair and enters him such that it is
smaller than a mustard seed and grows larger than mustard. Seeing as the mustard tree sees birds sitting on itself
and was the smallest of them all, what is its significance
other than what grows with age should enter us when we
are young, growing to such an extent that a human being
does not exist just for himself but also for all the others. In
this way, because human beings are to become trees and
fulfil this teaching of Christ and the example of the mustard tree — an old fully grown tree can no longer grasp
anything and is as good as dead in relation to the mustard
seed. Because he is dead and is nothing, and the example
refers to the mustard seed and not to the wood and
branches — how can a sprout grow out of an old pine? Or
from an old laurel a young elder? It is not possible. Even
more impossible is for an old proofreader in a printing
shop, an old convenor of an assembly of logicians, an old
father in a school to become a physician, because a physician should grow. How can the old ones still grow? They
have finished growing, have grown crooked and become
covered in moss so that nothing but knots and gnarls
remain. Hence, if a physician is to be firmly grounded he

must be sown in the cradle like a mustard seed and grow
in it like the great ones before God, like the Saints before
God, and must grow in such a way that in matters of medicine he grows like a mustard seed, that he grows beyond
all others. That must rise with youth and must grow.'
(Peuckert, Vol.1, p. 574f).

53. GA 79, p. 215.

54. GA 312, p. 182.

55. Like Paracelsus, Rudolf Steiner described this life-
sustaining nutritional process as a continuing struggle
against an inherently human consumption process. When
Paracelsus said: 'For a being resides in us which is like
fire; that same being gnaws away at our form and image.
... The consumption of form is fixed for the human being
as death. That self same death must be held at bay by the
human being through what nourishment does and is able
to do.' (Peuckert, Vol. 2, p. 32), then Rudolf Steiner says:
'You are continuously dying through the organization of
your 'I'; that is, you destroy your physical body internally
while in other respects external nature destroys your
physical body from the outside when you pass through
death. The physical body is capable of destruction from
two different directions and the organization of the 'I' is
simply the sum of destructive internal forces. It would
indeed be true to say that the organization of the 'I' has
the task of bringing about death ... which is always pre-
vented only in that there is new backup and this activity
of bringing about death only ever reaches the beginning
stages.' (GA 316, p. 30f.)

56. GA 303, p. 277.

57. GA 343, p. 42f.

58. GA 79, p. 211.

59. See Selg, *Vom Logos menschlicher Physis*. In particular pp.
199–215 and 489–504.

60. GA 343 (2), p. 66.

61. In this context we should take into account what Steiner
said with regard to the necessary transformation of *all* internalized substances — thus also of medicines: 'In reality,

there are not allopathic physicians, because those things, too, which are prescribed as allopathic medicines undergo a process of homoeopathy in the organism and in actual fact heal through the latter process. So that actually every allopathic physician finds support for his allopathic procedure through the homeopathic process in the patient's organism which actually undertakes what is omitted by the allopathic physician: the suspension of the interconnection of the individual parts of the medicine.' (GA 312, p.101). If Paracelsus — as described above — said with regard to the preparation of medicines that the earth substance had to be turned to 'chaos' for the cosmic influence to work, that is, had to suspended its inherent laws, Steiner used this concept also with regard to the human conception process in exactly the same way: 'The fertilized gamete is direct chaos with regard to the material, chaos which disintegrates, chaos which really disintegrates.' (GA 207, p. 128.) Only in this way does the egg cell open, or reopen itself to the 'pheripheral cosmic influences' (GA 343, p. 175) which determine embryonic development on a sustained basis.

62. GA 327, p. 23.
63. GA 346, p. 133.
64. GA 227, p. 108.
65. GA 227, p. 108. Maybe what Rudolf Steiner repeatedly described as the continuing development of *form* of the physical organs through breathing must be seen in this context: 'In the inhalation process, the human being is constantly being built up from the outside world and human beings really do not simply absorb the amorphous oxygen, but in the oxygen, which they mistakenly perceive as being amorphous, they take in the formative forces in accordance with their being. ... A developing human birth, a birth from the air into the human being is continuously happening from the macrocosm.' (GA 318, p. 97 and Selg, *Vom Logos menschlicher Physis*, pp. 512ff). We also refer here to the fundamental proximity of this statement to Paracelsus' description of the constant maintenance of form in the process of extended nutrition.

66. See GA 346, p. 137.

67. GA 343, p. 44

68. GA 343, p. 122.

69. GA 343, p. 260.

70. GA 344, p. 143.

71. GA 344, p. 146.

72. GA 344, p. 181.

73. GA 344, p. 181. That the action of the sacrificial offering of bread and wine is associated with the human *heart* (as organ of destiny, see p. 121) is already indicated in the Psalm in which it says: 'Thou dost cause the grass to grow for the cattle, and herbs for man to cultivate, and he may bring forth *food* from the earth, and *wine* to gladden the *heart* of man, oil to make his face shine, and *bread* to strengthen man's *heart*.' (Psalm 104:14f RSV, my emphasis). Compare in this respect also the statement by Paracelsus, already mentioned, that the sacramental food of Christ is preserved in the human *heart* where it grows.

74. GA 344, p. 149.

75. In this respect see particularly Steiner's account of July 15, 1914 in which he said: 'The guilt we accrue, the sin we accrue is not just a fact related to us — we have to make a distinction here — but it is an objective fact in the world, it is something that affects the world. We make up in our karma for deeds we have committed; but that we stabbed somebody's eyes out, for example, is a real event and if we, let us say, stab somebody's eyes out in this incarnation and then do something in the next to make up for that, it nevertheless remains in existence in terms of objective world events that we stabbed somebody's eyes out so and so many hundred years ago. That is an objective fact in the totality of the world. ... We must distinguish between the consequences of a sin for ourselves and the consequences of a sin for the objective progress of the world. ... We would have to bear unspeakable suffering if a being had not united with the earth which undoes those things for the earth which we ourselves can no longer change. This being

is Christ. He has taken the burden off us not of subjective karma, but of the spiritually objective effects of deeds, of guilt.' (GA 155, p. 183).

76. GA 343, p. 463. Even in his early lectures on earth and human history Steiner repeatedly said that the phenomenon of 'original sin' — as a (relative) connection between the human being and his hereditary relationships — has as an underlying factor the cosmic influences of adversary powers which want to force human beings to incarnate more deeply, thus exposing them to hereditary influences. This process, certainly constitutionally and psychologically significant, was not subject to human freedom (which did not yet exist as the result of insufficient ego development) and was only morally interpreted in later periods. See, for instance, GA 184, pp. 238ff.

77. GA 155, p. 157.

78. GA 169, p. 42.

79. With regard to the healing significance of the rhythmical centre of the human being, compare Steiner's lecture of April 13, 1921 (in GA 313) as well as the many references in the educational lectures in which Steiner described the healthy second year of life as the phase in which the rhythmical system dominates. That such overcoming of the pathological polarity between the nervous and sensory system and the metabolic and limb system implies the struggle of Christ with Lucifer and Ahriman at an existential level is dealt with in detail on p. 66f.

80. Selg, *Vom Logos menschlicher Physis,* pp. 687ff, 692.

81. GA 343, p. 605f.

82. GA 343, p. 248.

83. GA 268, p. 302.

4.The Soul Quickens in the Shrine of the Heart

1. GA 40, p.307.

2. See illustration in Zeylmans van Emmichoven, *Wer war Ita Wegman,* Vol. I.

3. GA 239, p. 31 and GA 128, p. 29.

4. GA 319, p. 171.

5. *Beiträge zur Rudolf Steiner Gesamtausgabe*, No. 16, Dornach 1966/67, p. 20.
6. GA 74, p. 93.
7. GA 212, p. 124.
8. GA 212, p. 127.
9. GA 205, p. 105.
10. GA 205, p. 111.
11. GA 205, p. 105.
12. Selg, *Vom Logos menschlicher Physis*, p. 688.
13. Selg, *Vom Logos menschlicher Physis*, p. 109 f.
14. In interpreting this quote from the gospels, Gerhard Kienle continued: 'where your heart is there will your eternal destiny be' *(Die ungeschriebene Philosophie Jesu*, p. 95). Kienle also pointed out, using the example of further quotes from the gospels, that the 'heart' in the gospels is the name for the 'centre of the soul' — 'almost what St Augustin and Fichte call "I"' (p. 94). Rudolf Steiner drew attention to this as well in 1909 when talking about Matthew 12:34 *(ex abundatia enim cordis os loquitur* 'When the mouth speaks, it reveals what is in the heart'): '"Heart" here stands for "I".' Compare Rudolf Steiner, GA 114, p. 188.
15. Written for Johanna Mücke on 29.10.1924. GA 268, p. 108
16. GA 26, p. 62.
17. GA 130, p. 92f.
18. See also the impressive account by Schöffler, 'Das Herz als Sinnesorgan bei Aristoteles und Thomas von Aquino' (The Heart as sensory organ in Aristotle and Thomas Aquinas) in *Die Zeitgestalt des Herzens*, pp. 70ff.

Bibliography

Benjamin, Walter, *Das Passagenwerk,* Frankfurt 1982.

Bock, Emil, *Die Drei Jahre* [The Three Years] Stuttgart 1998.

—, *Das Neue Testament,* Stuttgart 1987.

—, *The Three Years,* Edinburgh 1986.

Degenaar, A.G. *Krankheitsfälle und andere medizinische Fragen besprochen mit Dr Rudolf Steiner,* Stuttgart, no date.

Deggeller, Gerhard (ed.) *Paracelsus – Das Mahl der Herrn und Auslegung des Vaterunsers,* Dornach 1993.

Deventer, Madeleine P. van, *Die anthroposophisch-medizinische Bewegung in den verschiedenen Etappen ihrer Entwicklung,* Arlesheim 1992.

Fant, Ake, Klingborg, Arne & Wilkes, John A. *Die Holzplastik Rudolf Steiners in Dornach,* Dornach 1981.

Fiechter, Nik, 'Eine Heilmeditation für ein Kind' in *Mitteilungen aus der antrhoposophischen Arbeit in Deutschland,* 131/1980.

Frieling, Rudolf, *Christologische Aufsätze,* Stuttgart 1982.

Gaiser, Konrad, *Platons ungeschriebene Lehre,* Stuttgart 1962.

Hublow, Karl, *The Working of Christ in Man,* Edinburgh 1979.

Hublow, Karl & Joachim Krumbholz, *Heilung und Auferweckung,* [Working of Christ in Man] Stuttgart 1997.

Husemann, Gisbert, 'Lili Kolisko. Werk und Wesen' in *Beiträge zu einer Erweiterung der Heilkunst,* issue 2/1978, p. 38.

Kienle, Gerhard, *Christentum und Medizin,* Stuttgart 1986.

—, *Die Krankenpflege im Abendland,* in Selg, *Gerhard Kienle,* Vol. 2, pp.2321ff.

—, *Die ungeschriebene Philosophie Jesu,* Stuttgart 1986 (revised edition in Selg, *Gerhard Kienle,* Vol. 2, pp. 387ff.)

—, *Die Zeitlage im Verhältnis zu Raphael und Michael, in* Selg, *Gerhard Kienle,* Vol. 2, pp. 247ff.

Peuckert, Will-Erich (ed.) *Theophrastus Paracelsus. Werke,* Darmstadt 1965.

Pollock, S.J. 'Clinical trials. A practical approach,' quoted from Helmut Kiene, *Komplementäre Methodenlehre der klinischen Forschung. Cognition-based medicine.* Berlin, Heidelberg, New York 2000, p. 2.

Pörksen, Gunhild, 'Konturen des Ich – Paracelsus in Selbstzeugnissen,' in Dresdner Bombastus-Gesellschaft (ed.), *Erbe und Erben,* First Dresden Paracelsus Symposium, 28/29 December 1996.

Rittelmeyer, Friedrich, *Briefe über das Johannesevangelium,* Stuttgart 1947.

—, *Meine Lebensbegegnung mit Rudolf Steiner,* Stuttgart 1983.

Schöffler, Heinz Herbert, *Die Zeitgestalt des Herzens,* Stuttgart 1975.

Selg, Peter, *Anfänge anthroposophischer Heilkunst. Ita Wegman, Friedrich Husemann, Eugen Kolisko, F. Willem Zeylmans van Emmichoven, Karl König, Gerhard Kienle.* Pioniere der Anthroposophie, Dornach 2000.

— (ed.), *Anthroposophische Ärzte. Lebens- und Arbeitswege im 20. Jahrhundert. Nachrufe und Kurzbiographien,* Dornach 2000.

—, *Der Engel über dem Lauenstein. Siegfried Pickert, Ita Wegman und die Heilpädagogik,* Dornach 2004.

—, *Gerhard Kienle. Leben und Werk,* 2 volumes, Dornach 2003.

—, *Helene von Grunelius und Rudolf Steiners Kurse für junge Mediziner,* Dornach 2003.

—, *Krankheit, Heilung und Schicksal des Menschen. Über Rudolf Steiners geisteswissenschaftliches Pathologie und Therapieverständnis,* Dornach 2004.

—, *Vom Logos menschlicher Physis. Die Entfaltung einer anthroposophischen Humanphysiologie im Werk Rudolf Steiners,* Dornach 2000.

—, 'Die Medizin im Lebensgang Rudolf Steiners' in *Der Merkurstab,* issue 6/2000, pp. 377ff.

—, *Mysterium cordis. Studien zu einer sakramentalen Physiologie des Herzorgans,* Dornach 2003.

—, 'Die Paracelsus-Rezeption Rudolf Steiners' in *Mitteilungen aus der anthroposophischen Arbeit in Deutschland,* issue 215 (Easter 2001), p. 1–13.

Steiner, Rudolf, GA 26, *Anthroposophische Leitsätze* [Anthroposophical Leading Thoughts] Dornach 1989.

—, GA 28, *Mein Lebensgang* [Autobiography. Chapters from the Course of My Life] Dornach 1982.

—, GA 40, *Wahrspruchworte,* Dornach 1998.

—, GA 74, *Die Philosophie des Thomas von Aquino* [The Redemption of Thinking] Dornach 1967.

—, GA 79, *Die Wirklichkeit der höheren Welten,* Dornach 1988.

—, GA 100, *Menschheitsentwicklung und Christus-Erkenntnis,* Dornach 1981.

—, GA 107, *Geisteswissenschaftliche Menschenkunde,* Dornach 1988.

—, GA 112, *Das Johannes-Evangelium im Verhältnis zu den drei anderen Evangelien* [The Gospel of St John and Its Relation to the Other Gospels] Dornach 1984.

—, GA 114, *Das Lukas-Evangelium* [The Gospel of St Luke] Dornach 1985.

—, GA 116, *Der Christus-Impuls und die Entwicklung des Ich-Bewußtsein,* Dornach 1982.

—, GA 120, *Die Offenbarung des Karma* [Manifestation of Karma] Dornach 1975.

—, GA 123, *Das Matthäus-Evangelium* [The Gospel of St Matthew] Dornach 1988.

—, GA 125, *Wege und Ziele des geistigen Menschen,* Dornach 1978.

—, GA 128, *Eine okkulte Physiologie* [Occult Physiology] Dornach 1991.

—, GA 130, *Das esoterische Christentum und die geistige Führung der Menschheit,* Dornach 1987.

—, GA 131, *Von Jesus zu Christus* [From Jesus to Christ] Dornach 1988.

—, GA 133, *Der irdische und der kosmische Mensch,* Dornach 1989.

—, GA 139, *Das Markus-Evangelium* [The Gospel of St Mark] Dornach 1985.

—, GA 143, *Erfahrung des Übersinnlichen. Die Drei Wege der Seele zu Christus,* Dornach 1994.

—, GA 145, *Welche Bedeutung hat die okkulte Entwicklung des Menschen für seine Hüllen und sein Selbst?* Dornach 1986.

—, GA 150, *Die Welt des Geistes und ihr Hereinragen in das physische Dasein,* Dornach 1980.

—, GA 155, *Christus und die menschliche Seele*, Dornach 1994.

—, GA 156, *Okkultes Lesen und okkultes Hören*, Dornach 1987.

—, GA 158, *Der Zusammenhang des Menschen mit der elementarischen Welt*, Dornach 1993.

—, GA 169, *Weltwesen und Ichheit* [Cosmic Being and Egohood] Dornach 1963.

—, GA 170, *Das Rätsel des Menschen*, Dornach 1992.

—, GA 177, *Die spirituellen Hintergründe der äußeren Welt. Der Sturz der Geister der Finsternis*, Dornach 1987.

—, GA 178, *Individuelle Geisteswesen und ihr Wirken in der Seele des Menschen*, Dornach 1974.

—, GA 184, *Die Polarität von Dauer und Entwicklung im Menschen*, Dornach 1983.

—, GA 191, *Soziales Verständnis aus geisteswissenschaftlicher Erkenntnis* [The Influences of Lucifer and Ahriman] Dornach 1989.

—, GA 203, *Die Verantwortung des Menschen für die Weltentwicklung*, Dornach 1989.

—, GA 205, *Menschenwesen, Weltenseele und Weltengeist*, Part 1, Dornach 1987.

—, GA 207, *Anthroposophie als Kosmosophie I* [Cosmosophy] Dornach 1977.

—, GA 210, *Alte und neue Einweihungsmethoden*, Dornach 1967.

—, GA 211, *Das Sonnenmysterium und das Mysterium von Tod und Auferstehung*, Dornach 1986.

—, GA 212, *Menschliches Seelenleben und Geistesstreben*, Dornach 1978.

—, GA 216, *Die Grundimpulse des weltgeschichtlichen Werdens der Menschheit*, Dornach 1988.

—, GA 218, *Geistige Zusammenhänge in der Gestaltung des menschlichen Organismus*, Dornach 1976.

—, GA 227, *Initiationserkenntnis* [The Evolution of Consciousness] Dornach 1982.

—, GA 230, *Der Mensch als Zusammenklang der schaffenden, bildenden und gestaltenden Weltenwortes* [Man as Symphony of the Creative Word] Dornach 1970.

—, GA 238, *Esoterische Betrachtungen karmischer Zusammenhänge* [Karmic Relationships] Vol. 4, Dornach 1991.

—, GA 239, *Esoterische Betrachtungen karmischer Zusammenhänge* [Karmic Relationships. Esoteric Studies] Vol. 5, Dornach 1963.

—, GA 254, *Die okkulte Bewegung in neunzehnten Jahrhundert und ihre Beziehung zur Weltkultur* [The Occult Movement in the Nineteenth Century] Dornach 1986.

—, GA 266, *Menschenwesen, Menschenschicksal und Weltentwicklung,* Dornach 1988.

—, GA 260, *Die Weihnachtstagung* [The Christmas Conference] Dornach 1994.

—, GA 268, *Mantrische Sprüche. Seelenübungen II 1903-1925,* Dornach 1999.

—, GA 303, *Die gesunde Entwicklung des Menschenwesens* [Soul Economy and Waldorf Education] Dornach 1978.

—, GA 312, *Geistewissenschaft und Medizin* [Spiritual Science and Medicine] Dornach 1985.

—, GA 313, *Geisteswissenschaftliche Gesichtspunkte zur Therapie,* Dornach 1984.

—, GA 314, *Physiologisch-Therapeutisches auf Grundlage der Geisteswissenschaft,* Dornach 1989.

—, GA 316, *Meditative Anleitungen und Betrachtungen zur Vertiefung der Heilkunst,* Dornach 1987.

—, GA 317, *Heilpädagogischer Kurs,* (Education for Special Needs) Dornach 1987.

—, GA 318, *Pastoralmedizinischer Kurs* [Pastoral Medicine] Dornach 1994.

—, GA 319, *Anthroposophische Menschenerkenntnis und Medizin,* Dornach 1982.

—, GA 325, *Die Naturwissenschaft und die weltgeschichtliche Entwickelung der Menschheit seit dem Alterrum,* Dornach 1966.

—, GA 327, *Geisteswissenschaftliche Grundlagen zum Gedeihen der Landwirtschaft* [Agriculture] Dornach 1984.

—, GA 343, *Vorträge und Kurse über christlich-religiöses Wirken,* Vol. 2, Dornach 1993.

—, GA 344, *Vorträge und Kurse über christlich-religiöses Wirken,* Vol. 3, Dornach 1994.

—, GA 346, *Vorträge und Kurse über christlich-religiöses Wirken,* Vol. 5, [The Book of Revelation] Dornach 1995.

—, "Das Geheimnis der Wunde – Aufzeichnungen zum Samariterkurs" *Beiträge zur Rudolf Steiner Gesamtausgabe,* No. 108, Dornach 1992.

Steiner, Rudolf, and Wegman, Ita, *Grundlegendes zu einer Erweiterung der Heilkunst nach geisteswissenschaftlichen Erkenntnissen* [Extending Practical Medicine. Fundamental Principles Based on the Science of the Spirit] Dornach 1925.

Sudhoff, Karl (ed.) *Theophrast von Hohenheim, genannt Paracelsus. Sämtliche Werke.*

Walter, Hilma (ed.) *Im Anbruch der Wirkens für eine Erweiterung der Heilkunst. Die gesammelten Aufsätze aus "Natura" von Dr Ita Wegman,* Arlesheim 1974.

Wegman, Ita, *Das Mysterium der Erde.* In Walter, Hilma, *Im Anbruch der Wirkens für eine Erweiterung der Heilkunst.*

Zeylmans van Emmichoven, Emanuel, *Wer war Ita Wegman. Eine Dokumentation,* 3 volumes, Dornach 2000.

Zeylmans van Emmichoven, Emanuel, *Willem Zeylmans van Emmichoven,* Arlesheim 1979.